AF614690

Epidemiological and Clinico-Pathological Factors of COVID-19 in Children

Edited by Öner Özdemir

Published in London, United Kingdom

Epidemiological and Clinico-Pathological Factors of COVID-19 in Children
http://dx.doi.org/10.5772/intechopen.104347
Edited by Öner Özdemir

Contributors
Nicolás Padilla-Raygoza, Gilberto Flores-Vargas, María de Jesús Gallardo-Luna, Efrain Navarro-Olivos, Guadalupe Irazú Morales-Reyes, Jessica Paola Plascencia-Roldán, Kevin M. Kover, Moleboheng Emily Binyane, Polo-Ma-Abiele Hildah Mfengwana, Sherine Abdelmissih, Öner Özdemir, Emine Aylin Yılmaz

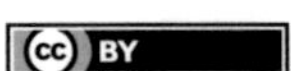

First published in London, United Kingdom, 2023 by IntechOpen
IntechOpen is the global imprint of INTECHOPEN LIMITED, registered in England and Wales, registration number: 11086078, 5 Princes Gate Court, London, SW7 2QJ, United Kingdom

British Library Cataloguing-in-Publication Data
A catalogue record for this book is available from the British Library

Additional hard and PDF copies can be obtained from orders@intechopen.com

Epidemiological and Clinico-Pathological Factors of COVID-19 in Children
Edited by Öner Özdemir
p. cm.
Print ISBN 978-1-80356-746-4
Online ISBN 978-1-80356-747-1
eBook (PDF) ISBN 978-1-80356-748-8

For EU product safety concerns:
IN TECH d.o.o., Prolaz Marije Krucifikse Kozulić 3, 51000 Rijeka, Croatia,
info@intechopen.com or visit our website at intechopen.com.

Meet the editor

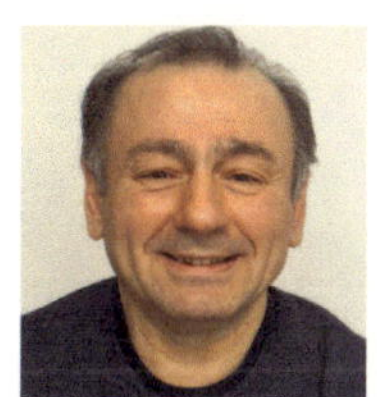

Prof. Dr. Öner Özdemir graduated from İstanbul Medical School, İstanbul University, Türkiye, and became a medical doctor in 1989. He completed his pediatric residency in the Department of Pediatrics, Children's Hospital, İstanbul Medical School, Türkiye. He completed his clinical fellowship training at the Pediatric Allergy/Immunology Division, Louisiana State University, Health Sciences Centre, USA. Some part of his clinical fellowship training was done at the Pediatric Allergy/Immunology program, Cincinnati Children's Hospital Medical Center, USA. Dr. Özdemir was the first-place winner of the 2005 Clemens Von Pirquet Award from the American College of Allergy, Asthma and Immunology (ACAAI) for the best research on allergy/asthma/immunology by a fellow in training. Dr. Özdemir has more than 250 national and international publications, more than 400 national and international presentations, and more than 20 book chapters to his credit. Dr. Özdemir has also edited seven books.

Contents

Preface IX

Section 1
Introduction 1

Chapter 1 3
Introductory Chapter: The Importance of COVID-19 Epidemiology in Children
by Öner Özdemir

Section 2
Ethio-Pathogenetic Factors 7

Chapter 2 9
SARS-CoV-2 Angiotensin Converting Enzyme 2 (ACE2) Receptor Expression and Its Effects on COVID-19 Epidemiology in Children
by Kevin M. Kover

Section 3
Epidemiology 21

Chapter 3 23
A Review on the Prevalence, Risk Factors, and Management of COVID-19 Disease in South African Children in Comparison to the World
by Moleboheng Emily Binyane and Polo-Ma-Abiele Hildah Mfengwana

Chapter 4 35
Epidemiology of SARS-CoV-2 Infection in Mexico and Latin America
by Nicolás Padilla-Raygoza, Gilberto Flores-Vargas, María de Jesús Gallardo-Luna, Efraín Navarro-Olivos, Guadalupe Irazú Morales-Reyes and Jessica Paola Plascencia-Roldán

Chapter 5 45
COVID-19 Epidemiology in Türkiye
by Emine Aylin Yılmaz and Öner Özdemir

Section 4
Clinico-Pathological Factors **53**

Chapter 6 **55**
4-Hydroxynonenal Is Linked to Sleep and Cognitive Disturbances in Children: Once upon the Time of COVID-19
by Sherine Abdelmissih

Preface

This book includes six chapters organized into four sections: "Introduction", "Ethio-Pathogenetic Factors", "Epidemiology," and "Clinico-Pathological Factors".

In Section 1, Chapter 1 discusses the importance of COVID-19 epidemiology in children. Knowing the factors that play a role in the epidemiology of this disease will help us to develop measures against them in possible future endemics and/or pandemic conditions.

In Section 2, Chapter 2 examines the role of angiotensin-converting enzyme 2 (ACE2) receptor expression in SARS-CoV-2 and its effects on COVID-19 epidemiology in children. The role and importance of ACE2 expression in the involvement of SARS-CoV-2 infection and COVID-19 disease has always been a point of discussion since the beginning of the pandemic.

In Section 3, Chapters 3–5 investigate the prevalence of COVID-19 in South Africa, Mexico, and Türkiye compared to other countries in the world, risk factors and changes in the care/treatment of the disease, and innovations and country-dependent approaches. The chapters give examples of pandemic prevention studies, treatment modalities, and vaccination studies developed according to the conditions of the regions discussed.

In Section 4, Chapter 6 discusses the link between 4-hydroxynonenal (HNE) and sleep and cognitive disturbances in children with COVID-19. Protein adducts of 4-hydroxynonenaline, a product of lipid peroxidation, have recently been investigated in studies of fatality in patients with COVID-19. Due to its relevance to the oxidant–antioxidant system, it can vary dynamically in the body in cases such as severe infection and chronic inflammation.

I would like to thank Publishing Process Manager Karla Skuliber and the staff at IntechOpen for their assistance throughout the publication process. I would also like to thank my wife Seval Hülya Özdemir and my daughter Berrin Nikame Özdemir for their support during the preparation of this book.

Öner Özdemir, MD
Division of Allergy and Immunology,
Department of Pediatrics,
Sakarya University Medical Faculty,
Research and Training Hospital,
Adapazarı, Sakarya, Türkiye

Section 1

Introduction

Chapter 1

Introductory Chapter: The Importance of COVID-19 Epidemiology in Children

Öner Özdemir

1. Introduction

In this book, apart from the section on the pathogenesis of COVID-19 disease, the factors that play a role in the etiology of the disease in different countries will be evaluated.

2. Discussion

The role of the renin-angiotensin system (RAS) in the pathogenesis of COVID-19 has been known from the beginning. The disproportion between angiotensin II (Ang II) and angiotensin1–7 (Ang1,7) occurred by the interplay between SARS-CoV-2 and angiotensin-converting enzyme 2 (ACE2) receptors is very important on the clinical table and prognosis. Other angiotensinases such as PRCP (prolyl carboxypeptidases) and POP (prolyl oligopeptidase) can lessen the deleterious effects of interplays between ACE2 and spike proteins of SARS-CoV-2. The deficiency of counter-regulatory RAS mechanisms in the acute phase of COVID-19 is presented by a decline in ACE2 expression due to unaffected activity of other angiotensinases and cannot prevent Ang II accumulation. Again, COVID-19 vaccines augment the endogenous synthesis of SARS-CoV-2 spike proteins. Therefore, unwanted effects of COVID-19 vaccination linked with Ang II buildup occur. Comprehension of the associations between the diverse mechanisms of Ang II degradation and buildup provides a chance to understand the pathophysiological cycle between the risk of development to severe types of COVID-19 disease and the possible unwanted effects of COVID-19 vaccination [1].

A zoonotic virus that causes severe respiratory diseases, three major outbreaks of the coronavirus including SARS-CoV, MERS-CoV, and most lately SARS-CoV-2, has been reported since 2002. Over the past few decades, the virus has been capable of mutating and changing, causing it to bypass the animal-to-human species barricade and infect humans. The appearance of SARS-CoV-2 created a serious global public health threat and caused major pandemic outbreaks. The latest pandemic of COVID-19, a disorder produced by SARS-CoV-2, in Wuhan, China's Hubei Province, has diseased more than 690 million people worldwide and caused fatality more than 6.8 million lives as of June 18, 2023. It has infected 213 other countries/regions worldwide. The virus constantly evolves and changes and spreads through asymptomatic carriers [2].

Epidemiologically, elderly individuals and people with predominant comorbidities are highly susceptible to grave health effects of COVID-19, comprising of cytokine upregulation and acute respiratory distress syndrome (ARDS) [3].

Multiple variants of the SARS-CoV-2 are known worldwide. This book discusses the overall picture of the pandemic in Latin America and several other countries, including its most common variants, how they affect surveillance at the genomic level, and the epidemiology of the disease. Again, the effect of COVID-19 vaccinations in Latin America and other countries on the epidemiology of the disease and how it can help alleviate the pandemic were also evaluated [4].

On March 5, 2020, South Africa registered its first imported patient of COVID-19. Since then, patients in South Africa have augmented exponentially with noteworthy communal spread. The situation in South Africa is also discussed in detail in our book [5].

A chapter in our book deals with the link of 4-hydroxynonenal (HNE) with sleep and cognitive disorders due to COVID-19 in children. As is known, protein adducts of the lipid peroxidation produce HNE was also found to be greater in the plasma of cases who died from the disease, while the total antioxidant capability was lower than the detection limit for most of the serum specimens. This suggests that the patients have active oxidative stress reaction mechanisms that respond to COVID-19 aggression. This may enable options to use antioxidants with a tailored, integrative biomedicine method to avert the initiation of a vicious cycle of HNE-mediated lipid peroxidation in cases with aggressive inflammatory disorders such as COVID-19 [6].

3. Conclusion

We hope that this book will help to understand the effects of lipid peroxidation elements such as HNE, which are little known, on the clinical picture, as well as their effects on the etiopathogenesis *via* the ACE-2 receptor, which is well known about COVID-19 disease.

Author details

Öner Özdemir
Division of Allergy and Immunology, Department of Pediatrics, Sakarya University Medical Faculty, Research and Training Hospital, Adapazarı, Sakarya, Türkiye

*Address all correspondence to: ozdemir_oner@hotmail.com

References

[1] Angeli F, Reboldi G, Trapasso M, Zappa M, Spanevello A, Verdecchia P. COVID-19, vaccines and deficiency of ACE2 and other angiotensinases. Closing the loop on the "Spike effect". European Journal of Internal Medicine. 2022;**103**:23-28. DOI: 10.1016/j.ejim.2022.06.015

[2] Sharma A, Ahmad Farouk I, Lal SK. COVID-19: A review on the novel coronavirus disease evolution, transmission, detection, control and prevention. Viruses. 2021;**13**(2):202. DOI: 10.3390/v13020202

[3] Muralidar S, Ambi SV, Sekaran S, Krishnan UM. The emergence of COVID-19 as a global pandemic: Understanding the epidemiology, immune response and potential therapeutic targets of SARS-CoV-2. Biochimie. 2020;**179**:85-100. DOI: 10.1016/j.biochi.2020.09.018

[4] García-López R, Laresgoiti-Servitje E, Lemus-Martin R, Sanchez-Flores A, Sanders-Velez C. The new SARS-CoV-2 variants and their epidemiological impact in Mexico. MBio. 2022;**13**(5):e0106021. DOI: 10.1128/mbio.01060-21

[5] Moonasar D, Pillay A, Leonard E, Naidoo R, Mngemane S, Ramkrishna W, et al. COVID-19: lessons and experiences from South Africa's first surge. BMJ Global Health. 2021;**6**(2):e004393. DOI: 10.1136/bmjgh-2020-004393

[6] Žarković N, Orehovec B, Milković L, Baršić B, Tatzber F, Wonisch W, et al. Preliminary findings on the association of the lipid peroxidation product 4-hydroxynonenal with the lethal outcome of aggressive COVID-19. Antioxidants (Basel). 2021;**10**(9):1341. DOI: 10.3390/antiox10091341

Section 2

Ethio-Pathogenetic Factors

Chapter 2

SARS-CoV-2 Angiotensin Converting Enzyme 2 (ACE2) Receptor Expression and Its Effects on COVID-19 Epidemiology in Children

Kevin M. Kover

Abstract

Children account for less than 2% of COVID-19 cases around the globe, and children experience relatively minor symptoms compared to the adult population. Various theories have been proposed to explain this phenomenon. One such theory is the involvement of angiotensin converting enzyme 2 (ACE2) in the pathogenesis of COVID-19. Previous studies have found a direct relationship between the abundance of pulmonary ACE2 receptors and the age of patients. Since Severe Acute Respiratory Syndrome Coronavirus 2 (SARS-CoV-2) binds to the ACE2 receptor to infect a patient, it is hypothesized that the low abundance of pulmonary ACE2 receptors in children relative to adults accounts for both the mild symptoms experienced as well as the difference in the number of identified cases.

Keywords: COVID-19, ACE2, RAAS, SARS, children, epidemiology, cases

1. Introduction

The World Health Organization (WHO) declared a global pandemic in March 2020 as COVID-19, an illness caused by SARS-CoV-2, was spreading rapidly around the globe, causing severe illness and death. There are numerous theories regarding the pathogenesis of COVID-19; however, it's pathogenesis is not completely understood due to the novelty of SARS-CoV-2. Various studies have been performed to determine how SARS-CoV-2 infects human cells so we can better understand its pathogenesis and, therefore, potential targets for medications and effective immunizations. COVID-19 is less prevalent in children than adults, accounting for less than 2% of cases. A few studies have demonstrated the potential involvement of ACE2, a component of the renin-angiotensin-aldosterone system (RAAS), as an explanation for the drastic difference between the number of COVID-19 cases in children versus adults. Multiple studies confirm that SARS-CoV-2 binds to ACE2, and there is a higher abundance of pulmonary ACE2 receptors in adults compared to children.

These two conclusions together could provide insight into the lower number of COVID-19 cases and the lower severity of symptoms in children.

2. The coronavirus disease (COVID-19)

In December 2019, pneumonia of an unknown origin was linked to a seafood wholesale market in Wuhan, Hubei Province, China. Scientists isolated a novel coronavirus related to SARS-CoV. Therefore, it was named SARS-CoV-2, and the disease that it causes was named coronavirus disease 2019 (COVID-19). This novel disease began to spread globally due to its high rate of infectivity. Because of the high rate of mortality caused by COVID-19, the WHO declared a global pandemic in March 2020 [1, 2]. As of November 2022, the total number of cases in the United States was 98,481,551 including 305,082 new cases. The total number of deaths due to COVID-19 was 1,075,779 as of November of 2022, including 2,644 new deaths, and the number of hospitalizations was 25,224 with an average of 3,915 new admissions daily [3].

On December 14, 2020, the U.S. COVID Vaccination Program began where vaccines from Pfizer, Moderna, and Johnson & Johnson were administered around the globe [4]. Pfizer and Moderna each initially required 2 shots to be fully immunized, whereas Johnson & Johnson required 1 shot [5]. At that time, Pfizer vaccines were given to patients ages 12 and older, while Moderna and Johnson & Johnson vaccines were given to patients ages 18 and older [5]. As of December 2022, Pfizer and Moderna vaccines were being offered to children as young as 6 months of age [6].

3. COVID-19 illness symptoms and severity in children

Like adults, COVID-19 infection in children can cause severe illness, especially if they have an underlying health condition such as congenital heart disease, asthma, type 1 diabetes, obesity, cystic fibrosis, cancer, or immunosuppression [7–9]. In rare circumstances, children with severe COVID-19 infection may develop a condition known as multisystem inflammatory syndrome in children (MIS-C) [8].

MIS-C is a severe post-infectious inflammatory complication of COVID-19 in children where most patients (about 68%) required mechanical ventilation and ICU admission. The most common presentation of MIS-C was gastrointestinal symptoms such as diarrhea and abdominal pain. The majority MIS-C cases demonstrated neutrophilia and an elevated inflammatory marker called c-reactive protein (CRP) [10]. MIS-C commonly affects children ages 5–13 and has been associated with coronary artery aneurysms, left ventricular cardiac dysfunction, atrioventricular block, and multiorgan failure [11, 12]. New evidence suggests MIS-C infection in neonates, now termed multisystem inflammatory syndrome in neonates (MIS-N) [11, 13–17]. As of November 28, 2022, the CDC reports 9,139 confirmed cases of MIS-C and 74 deaths. Half of these cases were children ages 5–13 years old with a median age of 9 years old. 98% of children tested positive for COVID-19; the remaining 2% were exposed to COVID-19 [18]. **Figures 1** and **2** demonstrate the weekly cases of MIS-C throughout the pandemic and the number of cases per age range, respectively.

Recent research regarding COVID-19 infection in children versus adults is controversial. Children often experience a milder course of illness or are asymptomatic [19, 20], making it difficult to establish the number of pediatric cases. Research has shown that a component of the RAAS, ACE2, has been linked to lower COVID-19 infection

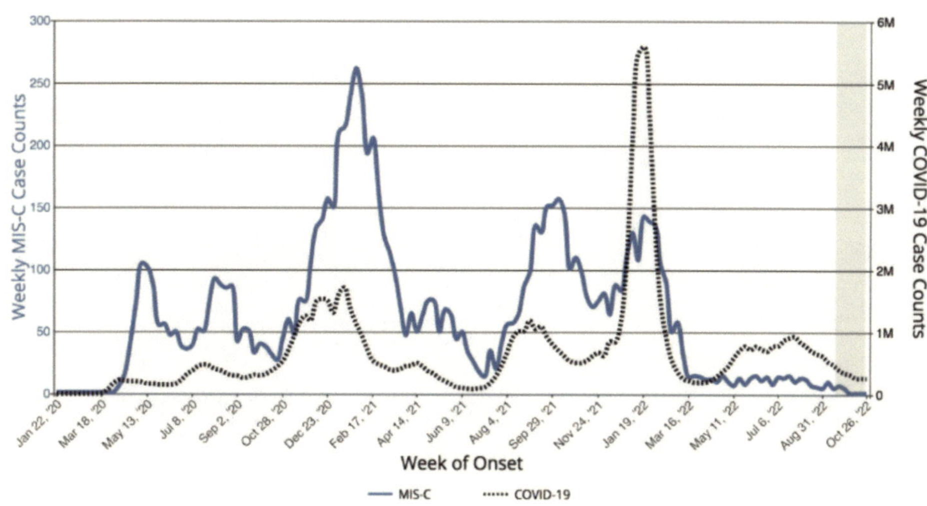

Figure 1.
Weekly MIS-C Cases and COVID-19 Cases Reported to CDC [18].

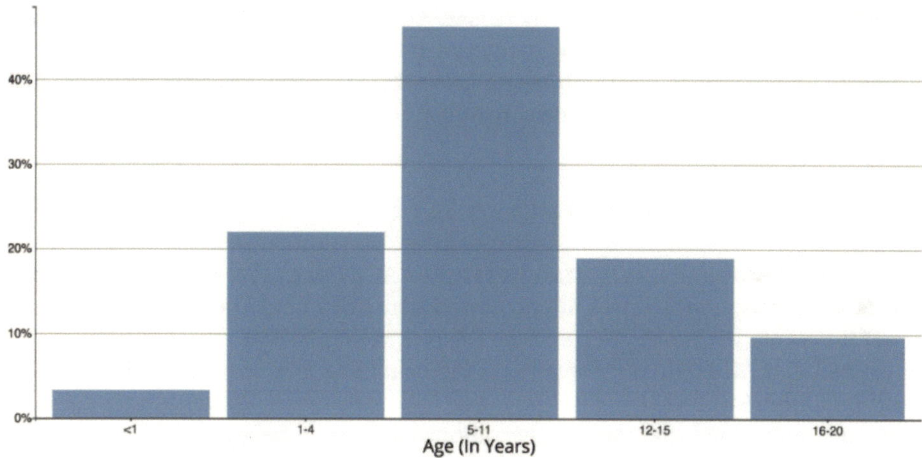

Figure 2.
MIS-C Patients by Age Group [18].

rates and milder symptoms of COVID-19 infection in the pediatric population compared to the adult population.

4. Renin-angiotensin-aldosterone system (RAAS)

Blood pressure is regulated by the kidneys via the RAAS. Juxtaglomerular (JG) cells in the kidney release renin, a protein that helps to increase blood pressure. A rise in blood pressure is accomplished when renin acts on angiotensinogen, which is released from the liver, to convert it into its active form, angiotensin I. Angiotensin I is then converted to angiotensin II via ACE in the lungs. Angiotensin II serves to increase blood pressure and blood volume by triggering the release of aldosterone and antidiuretic hormone (ADH). Aldosterone and ADH reabsorb sodium and water,

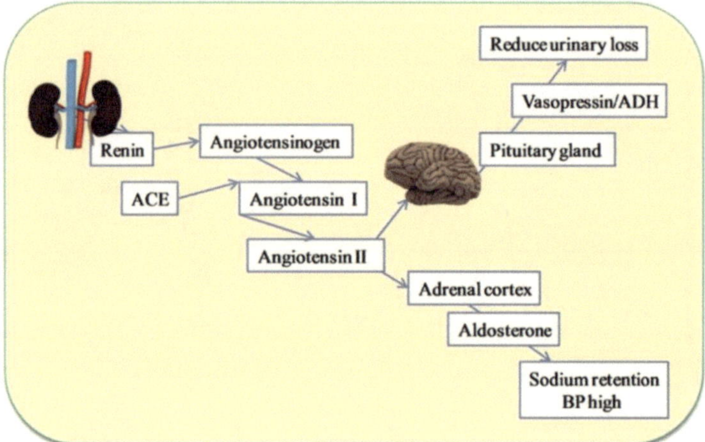

Figure 3.
Diagram of the RAAS [22].

respectively, from the kidney. As water follows sodium into the body, blood volume increases; therefore, blood pressure increases. Angiotensin II also causes vasoconstriction that leads to an increase in blood pressure. Because of these effects, classes of medications known as ACE inhibitors (ACEi) and angiotensin receptor blockers (ARB) can be used to manage the blood pressure of hypertensive patients (**Figure 3**) [21].

5. Biochemical comparison of ACE to ACE2

ACE2 was discovered in 2001 and was named ACE2 due to its structural similarity to ACE. Consequently, it was hypothesized that ACE2 could be another potential target for the treatment of hypertension. Despite its similarity to ACE, studies determined that ACE2 did not convert angiotensin I to angiotensin II, and ACEi were unable to inhibit ACE2 [23].

Studies determined that the major structural difference between ACE and ACE2 was that ACE is a carboxy-dipeptidase that removed C-terminal dipeptide, while ACE2 acted as a carboxy-peptidase that removed only a single amino acid. ACE2 hydrolyzes angiotensin I more poorly when compared to ACE; however, it was determined that ACE2 hydrolyzes angiotensin II with a catalytic efficacy of about 400-fold compared to ACE2 hydrolysis of angiotensin I [23, 24]. Originally, the main tissue sites that expressed ACE2 receptors were the testes, heart, and kidney [23, 25].

It is now known that ACE2 receptors are present in the respiratory tract, specifically the olfactory epithelium, the nasal septal epithelium, the nasal conchae, and the paranasal sinuses [26].

6. ACE2 and SARS-CoV-1

In 2003, a novel coronavirus known as SARS-CoV-1 [27] was identified as a distinct etiological agent for SARS [28–32]. SARS is known to be a lower respiratory tract disease, and numerous coronavirus particles were found in pneumocytes [32, 33], cells that are located in the alveoli of the lungs. Furthermore, a large number of

ACE2 receptors were found in type I and type II pneumocytes [32, 34], and few ACE2 receptors were discovered in the bronchial epithelium [32]. This evidence supports the hypothesis that SARS is likely linked to the ACE2 receptors as both were associated with each other in the alveoli.

The spike proteins of SARS-CoV-1 were found to target several ACE2 receptors located in various organs, including the immune system and respiratory tract, which can result in immunosuppression and respiratory distress, respectively. Therefore, it was concluded that SARS-CoV-1 was linked to the ACE2 receptor; consequently, ACE2 was hypothesized as a potential target for treatment of SARS.

7. ACE2 and SARS-CoV-2

As previously mentioned, recent research shows that ACE2 is linked to SARS-CoV-2. The binding affinity is vastly different due to amino acid differences at the biochemical level between ACE2 and ACE. There are stronger hydrophobic and salt bridge interactions between SARS-CoV-2 and ACE2 compared to those between SARS-CoV-2 and ACE. This was hypothesized as the explanation for the larger global influence COVID-19 has had compared to SARS-CoV-1 [35–37].

As stated above, the spike protein (S-protein) of SARS-CoV-2 and SARS-CoV-1 is what binds to the extracellular domains of ACE2 in the lungs. This leads to subsequent downregulation of ACE2 receptors which allows SARS-CoV-2 to be endocytosed into the cell it is infecting. ACE2 receptors have been found to protect the cells where they are expressed; therefore, their downregulation upon binding of SARS-CoV-2 is what allows endocytosis and subsequent COVID-19 infection [37–40]. **Figures 4** and **5** demonstrate the interactions between ACE2 and SARS-CoV-2 as well as the pathogenesis of COVID-19 and the human immune response.

The human immune system responds to the loss of ACE2 receptors via an imbalance of Th17 and Treg cell function leading to an overactivation of immune cells [37, 41–43]. The imbalance of the RAAS system along with ACE2 receptor loss in COVID-19 patients are additional factors that contribute to tissue and systemic inflammation [37, 44, 45].

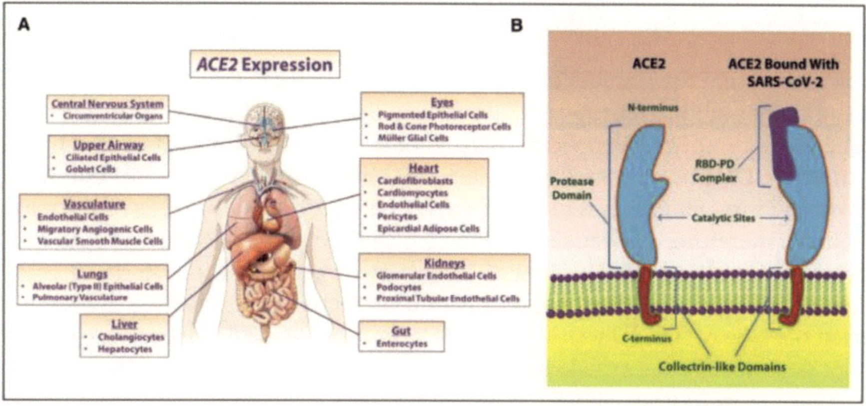

Figure 4.
Location of various organs that contain ACE2 receptors with their function (A) and ACE2 binding to SARS-CoV-2 (B) [37].

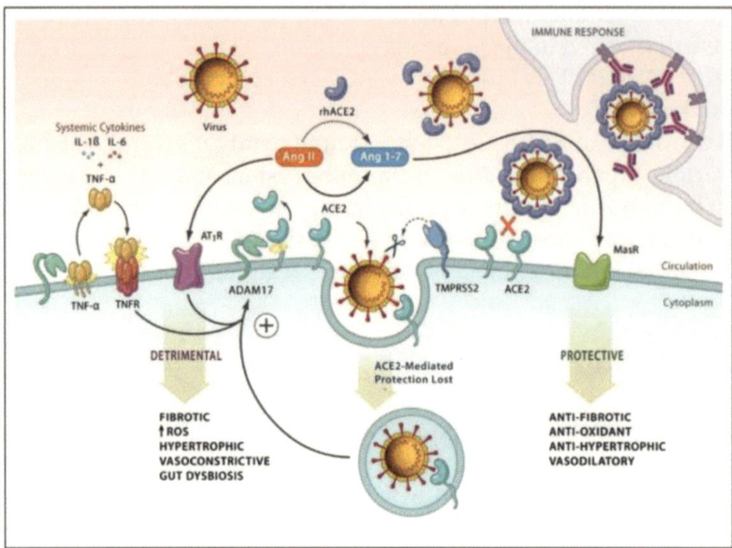

Figure 5.
Role of ACE2 in the pathogenesis of COVID-19 and the inflammatory response [37].

8. COVID-19 infection, children versus adults

As previously stated, the diagnosis of COVID-19 in children is more difficult than that of adults and can be controversial. This is because children who are infected with SARS-CoV-2 are often asymptomatic or mildly symptomatic; consequently, they are not typically tested for COVID-19. Anosmia and ageusia are not frequent in children, but when present, they are the strongest predictors of SARS-CoV-2 infection [46].

Data from the World Health Organization (WHO) from December 2019 to September 2021 showed that children under 5 represented 1.8% of global COVID-19 cases and 0.1% of global deaths. Children ages 5 to 14 years of age were 6.3% of global cases and 0.1% of global deaths [47, 48].

9. ACE2 receptor expression, children versus adults

It is known that the number of global COVID-19 cases in children is significantly less than that of adults. A proposed mechanism for this distribution is the hypothesis that the ACE2 receptor is expressed to a higher degree in the lungs of adults than it is in children. Data has shown that SARS-CoV-2 binds to ACE2 receptors before it is endocytosed into pneumocytes located deep in the lungs and into cells of the nasal epithelium; therefore, a lower expression of ACE2 receptors in children could explain the drastic difference in the number of cases between children and adults.

A 2020 retrospective study by Bunyavanich and colleagues involved 305 subjects between the ages of 4 to 60 years of age. They found that ACE2 receptor expression was age-dependent where the lowest number of ACE2 gene expression was found in children less than 10 years of age [49].

The number of ACE2 gene expression significantly increased as age increased [49]. Thus, the researchers proposed that this data could potentially explain why COVID-19 is less prevalent in children than in adults [49, 50].

Furthermore, it was previously mentioned that severe cases of COVID-19 in children, such as those seen in MIS-C and MIS-N, mainly exhibit gastrointestinal symptoms while severe cases in adults affect the pulmonary system more than the gastrointestinal system. A 2022 study by Schurink and colleagues found that as age increases, ACE2 receptor expression increases in the lungs and decreases in the intestines [51], which could explain why older individuals experience more severe pulmonary complications compared to children. Gastrointestinal issues in children can be caused by a variety of pathogens and can potentially be overlooked as a severe COVID-19 infection, which can also contribute to lower cases of COVID-19 cases in children.

10. Conclusion

The COVID-19 pandemic caused by SARS-CoV-2 has had a significant impact on the global population. Countless efforts have been made to decrease transmission of and eradicate the virus, including medications and vaccines. Several different studies have been performed to determine the pathogenesis of SARS-CoV-2 so we can better understand how it infects the population and to find targets for medications that can hopefully treat the infection and prevent severe illness.

Not only has COVID-19 significantly impacted the global population, but it has impacted children to a much lesser degree than adults with children representing less than 2% of global COVID-19 cases. A proposed mechanism for explaining why cases are much less prevalent in children is the lower expression of pulmonary ACE2 receptors, a component of the RAAS, in the nasal epithelium and alveolar pneumocytes of children compared to adults. Studies have shown that SARS-CoV-2 binds to ACE2 before being endocytosed into cells to cause infection. Studies also show the number of ACE2 receptors in the pulmonary system is directly related to age.

This proposed mechanism is controversial at this point in time, especially since COVID-19 cases in children may also be likely lower because they experience mildly symptomatic or asymptomatic illness. Future studies should involve compounds that specifically inhibit pulmonary ACE2 in adults to determine if the number of COVID-19 cases significantly decrease. Eventually, these developments can lead to medications to treat the virus at its early stages to decrease likelihood of transmission and, therefore, prevent severe illness.

Acknowledgements

I would like to express my sincere gratitude to Dr. Öner Özdemir for giving me the opportunity to contribute to his book: *COVID-19 Epidemiology in Children*. I would also like to thank the Sharpe Strumia Research Foundation at the Bryn Mawr Hospital at Main Line Health for funding this work. Lastly, I would like to recognize author service manager, Karla Skuliber, for her assistance in the completion of my chapter.

Author details

Kevin M. Kover
Main Line Health, Philadelphia, PA, USA

*Address all correspondence to: kevinkover@gmail.com

References

[1] Ciotti M, Ciccozzi M, Terrinoni A, Jiang WC, Wang CB, Bernardini S. The COVID-19 pandemic. Critical Reviews in Clinical Laboratory Sciences. 2020;**57**(6):365-388

[2] Czulada L, Kover KM, Gracias G, Kumar KN, Desai S, Stawicki SP, et al. Toxic stress affecting families and children during the COVID-19 pandemic: A global mental health crisis and an emerging international health security threat. In: Contemporary Developments and Perspectives in International Health Security. London, UK: IntechOpen; 2022

[3] Centers for Disease Control and Prevention. COVID Data Tracker [Internet]. Centers for Disease Control and Prevention. 2020. Available from: https://covid.cdc.gov/covid-data-tracker/#datatracker-home

[4] CDC. COVID Data Tracker Weekly Review [Internet]. Centers for Disease Control and Prevention. 2023 [cited 2023 Jan 13]. Available from: http://www.cdc.gov/coronavirus/2019-ncov/covid-data/covidview/index.html

[5] CDC. Different COVID-19 Vaccines [Internet]. Centers for Disease Control and Prevention. 2022. Available from: http://www.cdc.gov/coronavirus/2019-ncov/vaccines/different-vaccines.html

[6] CDC. COVID-19 Vaccination [Internet]. Centers for Disease Control and Prevention. 2022. Available from: https://www.cdc.gov/coronavirus/2019-ncov/vaccines/stay-up-to-date.html#children

[7] Woodruff RC, Campbell AP, Taylor CA, Chai SJ, Kawasaki B, Meek J, et al. Risk factors for severe COVID-19 in children. Pediatrics. Jan 2022;**149**(1):e2021053418

[8] CDC. COVID Data Tracker [Internet]. Centers for Disease Control and Prevention. 2020. Available from: https://covid.cdc.gov/covid-data-tracker/#pediatric-data

[9] CDC. COVID-19 and Your Health [Internet]. Centers for Disease Control and Prevention. 2020. Available from: https://www.cdc.gov/coronavirus/2019-ncov/need-extra-precautions/people-with-medical-conditions.html#MedicalConditionsAdults

[10] Radia T, Williams N, Agrawal P, Harman K, Weale J, Cook J, et al. Multi-system inflammatory syndrome in children & adolescents (MIS-C): A systematic review of clinical features and presentation. Paediatric Respiratory Reviews. 2021;**38**:51-57

[11] Molloy EJ, Nakra N, Gale C, Dimitriades VR, Lakshminrusimha S. Multisystem inflammatory syndrome in children (MIS-C) and neonates (MIS-N) associated with COVID-19: Optimizing definition and management. Pediatric Research. 2022;**2022**:1

[12] Nakra NA, Blumberg DA, Herrera-Guerra A, Lakshminrusimha S. Multi-system inflammatory syndrome in children (MIS-C) following SARS-CoV-2 infection: Review of clinical presentation, hypothetical pathogenesis, and proposed management. Children. 2020;**7**(7):69

[13] Pawar R, Gavade V, Patil N, Mali V, Girwalkar A, Tarkasband V, et al. Neonatal multisystem inflammatory syndrome (MIS-N) associated with prenatal maternal SARS-CoV-2: A case series. Children. 2021;**8**(7):572

[14] Divekar AA, Patamasucon P, Benjamin JS. Presumptive neonatal

multisystem inflammatory syndrome in children associated with coronavirus disease 2019. American Journal of Perinatology. 2021;**38**(06):632-636

[15] Diwakar K, Gupta BK, Uddin MW, Sharma A, Jhajra S. Multisystem inflammatory syndrome with persistent neutropenia in neonate exposed to SARS-CoV-2 virus: A case report and review of literature. Journal of Neonatal-Perinatal Medicine. 2022;**15**(2):373-377

[16] Diggikar S, Nanjegowda R, Kumar A, Kumar V, Kulkarni S, Venkatagiri P. Neonatal Multisystem Inflammatory Syndrome secondary to SARS-CoV-2 infection. Journal of Paediatrics and Child Health. May 2021;**58**(5):900

[17] More K, Aiyer S, Goti A, Parikh M, Sheikh S, Patel G, et al. Multisystem inflammatory syndrome in neonates (MIS-N) associated with SARS-CoV2 infection: A case series. European Journal of Pediatrics. 2022;**181**(5):1883-1898

[18] CDC. COVID Data Tracker [Internet]. Centers for Disease Control and Prevention. 2020. Available from: https://covid.cdc.gov/covid-data-tracker/#mis-national-surveillance

[19] CDC. Coronavirus Disease 2019 (COVID-19) [Internet]. Centers for Disease Control and Prevention. 2020. Available from: https://www.cdc.gov/coronavirus/2019-ncov/hcp/pediatric-hcp.html

[20] Martin B, DeWitt PE, Russell S, Anand A, Bradwell KR, Bremer C, et al. Characteristics, outcomes, and severity risk factors associated with SARS-CoV-2 infection among children in the US national COVID cohort collaborative. JAMA Network Open. 2022;**5**(2):e2143151

[21] Le T. First Aid for the Usmle Step 1. Norwalk: Mcgraw-Hill Educ Medical; 2015

[22] Patel S, Rauf A, Khan H, Abu-Izneid T. Renin-angiotensin-aldosterone (RAAS): The ubiquitous system for homeostasis and pathologies. Biomedicine & Pharmacotherapy. 2017;**94**:317-325

[23] Clarke NE, Turner AJ. Angiotensin-converting enzyme 2: The first decade. International Journal of Hypertension. Oct 2012;**2012**

[24] Burrell LM, Johnston CI, Tikellis C, Cooper ME. ACE2, a new regulator of the renin–angiotensin system. Trends in Endocrinology and Metabolism. 2004;**15**(4):166-169

[25] Tipnis SR, Hooper NM, Hyde R, Karran E, Christie G, Turner AJ. A human homolog of angiotensin-converting enzyme: Cloning and functional expression as a captopril-insensitive carboxypeptidase. The Journal of Biological Chemistry. 2000;**275**(43):33238-33243

[26] Klingenstein M, Klingenstein S, Neckel PH, Mack AF, Wagner AP, Kleger A, et al. Evidence of SARS-CoV2 entry protein ACE2 in the human nose and olfactory bulb. Cells, Tissues, Organs. 2020;**209**(4-6):155-164

[27] Rat P, Olivier E, Dutot M. SARS-CoV-2 vs. SARS-CoV-1 management: Antibiotics and inflammasome modulators potential. European Review for Medical and Pharmacological Sciences. 2020;**24**(14):7880-7885

[28] Ksiazek TG, Erdman D, Goldsmith CS, Zaki SR, Peret T, Emery S, et al. A novel coronavirus associated with severe acute respiratory syndrome. The New England Journal of Medicine. 2003;**348**(20):1953-1966

[29] Drosten C, Günther S, Preiser W, Van Der Werf S, Brodt HR, Becker S, et al.

Identification of a novel coronavirus in patients with severe acute respiratory syndrome. The New England Journal of Medicine. 2003;**348**(20):1967-1976

[30] Kuiken T, Fouchier RA, Schutten M, Rimmelzwaan GF, Van Amerongen G, Van Riel D, et al. Newly discovered coronavirus as the primary cause of severe acute respiratory syndrome. The Lancet. 2003;**362**(9380):263-270

[31] Fouchier RA, Kuiken T, Schutten M, Van Amerongen G, Van Doornum GJ, Van Den Hoogen BG, et al. Koch's postulates fulfilled for SARS virus. Nature. 2003;**423**(6937):240

[32] Hamming I, Timens W, Bulthuis ML, Lely AT, Navis GV, van Goor H. Tissue distribution of ACE2 protein, the functional receptor for SARS coronavirus. A first step in understanding SARS pathogenesis. The Journal of Pathology: A Journal of the Pathological Society of Great Britain and Ireland. 2004;**203**(2):631-637

[33] Ding Y, Wang H, Shen H, Li Z, Geng J, Han H, et al. The clinical pathology of severe acute respiratory syndrome (SARS): A report from China. The Journal of Pathology: A Journal of the Pathological Society of Great Britain and Ireland. 2003;**200**(3):282-289

[34] To KF, Tong JH, Chan PK, Au FW, Chim SS, Allen Chan KC, et al. Tissue and cellular tropism of the coronavirus associated with severe acute respiratory syndrome: An in-situ hybridization study of fatal cases. The Journal of Pathology: A Journal of the Pathological Society of Great Britain and Ireland. 2004;**202**(2):157-163

[35] Yan R, Zhang Y, Li Y, Xia L, Guo Y, Zhou Q. Structural basis for the recognition of SARS-CoV-2 by full-length human ACE2. Science. 2020;**367**(6485):1444-1448

[36] Shang J, Ye G, Shi K, Wan Y, Luo C, Aihara H, et al. Structural basis of receptor recognition by SARS-CoV-2. Nature. 2020;**581**(7807):221-224

[37] Gheblawi M, Wang K, Viveiros A, Nguyen Q, Zhong JC, Turner AJ, et al. Angiotensin-converting enzyme 2: SARS-CoV-2 receptor and regulator of the renin-angiotensin system: Celebrating the 20th anniversary of the discovery of ACE2. Circulation Research. Oct 2020;**126**(10):1456-1474

[38] Li W, Moore MJ, Vasilieva N, Sui J, Wong SK, Berne MA, et al. Angiotensin-converting enzyme 2 is a functional receptor for the SARS coronavirus. Nature. 2003;**426**(6965):450-454

[39] Walls AC, Park YJ, Tortorici MA, Wall A, McGuire AT, Veesler D. Structure, function, and antigenicity of the SARS-CoV-2 spike glycoprotein. Cell. 2020;**181**(2):281-292

[40] Zhou P, Yang XL, Wang XG, Hu B, Zhang L, Zhang W, et al. A pneumonia outbreak associated with a new coronavirus of probable bat origin. Nature. 2020;**579**(7798):270-273

[41] Imai Y, Kuba K, Rao S, Huan Y, Guo F, Guan B, et al. Angiotensin-converting enzyme 2 protects from severe acute lung failure. Nature. 2005;**436**(7047):112-116

[42] Kuba K, Imai Y, Ohto-Nakanishi T, Penninger JM. Trilogy of ACE2: A peptidase in the renin–angiotensin system, a SARS receptor, and a partner for amino acid transporters. Pharmacology & Therapeutics. 2010;**128**(1):119-128

[43] Jia H. Pulmonary angiotensin-converting enzyme 2 (ACE2) and inflammatory lung disease. Shock. 2016;**46**(3):239-248

[44] Zhou F, Yu T, Du R, Fan G, Liu Y, Liu Z, et al. Clinical course and risk factors for mortality of adult inpatients with COVID-19 in Wuhan, China: A retrospective cohort study. The Lancet. 2020;**395**(10229):1054-1062

[45] Wan Y, Shang J, Graham R, Baric RS, Li F. Receptor recognition by the novel coronavirus from Wuhan: An analysis based on decade-long structural studies of SARS coronavirus. Journal of Virology. 2020;**94**(7):e00127-e00120

[46] Nikolopoulou GB, Maltezou HC. COVID-19 in children: Where do we stand? Archives of Medical Research. 2022;**53**(1):1-8

[47] COVID-19 disease in children and adolescents: Scientific brief, 29 September 2021 [Internet]. www.who.int. Available from: https://www.who.int/publications-detail-redirect/WHO-2019-nCoV-Sci_Brief-Children_and_adolescents-2021.1

[48] Who.int. 2021. Available from: https://covid19.who.int/measures

[49] Bunyavanich S, Do A, Vicencio A. Nasal gene expression of angiotensin-converting enzyme 2 in children and adults. Journal of the American Medical Association. 2020;**323**(23):2427-2429

[50] Dong Y, Mo X, Hu Y, Qi X, Jiang F, Jiang Z, et al. Epidemiology of COVID-19 among children in China. Pediatrics. 2020;**145**(6)

[51] Schurink B, Roos E, Vos W, Breur M, van der Valk P, Bugiani M. ACE2 protein expression during childhood, adolescence, and early adulthood. Pediatric and Developmental Pathology. 2022;**2022**:1093

Section 3

Epidemiology

Chapter 3

A Review on the Prevalence, Risk Factors, and Management of COVID-19 Disease in South African Children in Comparison to the World

Moleboheng Emily Binyane
and Polo-Ma-Abiele Hildah Mfengwana

Abstract

The first case of coronavirus disease of 2019 (COVID-19) in South Africa (SA) was first reported at the beginning of March 2022, and then further spread from Gauteng, Western Cape, and KwaZulu Natal to the rest of the provinces. It is caused by severe acute respiratory syndrome coronavirus 2. In SA, COVID-19 is less prevalent in children less than 18 years. Only a few studies describe the epidemiology, risk factors, and clinical manifestation of COVID-19 among children in SA in comparison to other countries including China, North America, and Europe. South African children are affected by conditions including poverty, tuberculosis, and human immunodeficiency virus which predispose them to COVID-19. Overcrowding and limited healthcare facilities and resources also complicated the diagnosis and clinical and pharmacological management of COVID-19 in SA. The current review discusses the prevalence, risk factors, and management of COVID-19 in South African children in comparison to other continents in the world.

Keywords: COVID-19, epidemiology, children, management, South Africa

1. Introduction

The World Health Organization (WHO) reports that virus-causing diseases are still a serious public health issue [1]. Apart from the global pandemic caused by the severe acute respiratory syndrome coronavirus-2 (SARS-CoV-2), the twenty-first century has experienced a flood of viral infectious diseases [2]. The severe acute respiratory syndrome coronavirus outbreak occurred in 2003, followed by the 2009 swine flu pandemic, the Middle East respiratory syndrome coronavirus 2012 outbreak, the West Africa Ebola Virus disease epidemic between 2013 and 2016, and the 2015 Zika virus disease epidemic in various countries [2]. WHO declared the Coronavirus disease 2019 (COVID-19) a

IntechOpen

global emergency on January 30, 2020 [3]. The highly communicable respiratory disease COVID-19 is caused by SARS-CoV-2 belonging to the family Coronaviridae capable of causing infections in humans and vertebrate animals [4–6]. A bat is reported to be the natural host for SARS-CoV-2 but the pandemic-causing infections that occurred in humans were because of the intermediate host, the pangolin [7, 8]. The COVID-19 pandemic began in Wuhan, the capital of Hubei province, China on December 31, 2019 [8], and within five months had progressed worldwide and reached South Africa (SA) in March 2020 [8, 9]. Currently, there are a limited number of studies reporting on the epidemiology and clinical manifestations of COVID-19 in South African children [10]. However, most studies focus on children residing in China, Europe, Australia, North America, South America, Iran, and the Democratic Republic of Congo. Therefore, their findings might not be generalizable to SA due to the differences in risk factors predisposing children to COVID-19. Furthermore, identified risk factors in South African children include, human immunodeficiency virus (HIV), tuberculosis (TB), malnutrition, childhood obesity, overcrowding, and limited access to quality healthcare facilities for effective prevention and management of COVID-19 [10]. In SA, changes in the epidemiology of SARS-CoV-2 among children and adolescents less than 18 years in comparison to adults were reported [11]. During the first wave, the rates of infection were higher in infants, and the rates increased in all age groups during the second and third waves. However, significant changes were observed during the omicron BA.1/BA.2 wave where the number of infections dropped in individuals in less than one year and increased in those over one year [10]. These changes could be attributed to the variation in the population's immunity from natural infection, vaccination, and the characteristics and potential effects of the emerging variants on SARS-CoV-2-related illness in children [11]. SARS-CoV-2 infection in children is in most cases asymptomatic or causes milder symptoms than in adults, and as a result, children are less likely to be tested or receive clinical management [10, 12]. Other studies have reported that SARS-CoV-2-infected children can also be seriously ill and manifest the signs of the multisystem inflammatory syndrome in children such as persistent fever, severe gastrointestinal (GIT) symptoms, systemic excessive inflammation, multiple organ involvement, and symptoms like toxic shock syndrome (TSS) [13]. Treatment of COVID-19 in children includes supportive care and pharmacological management with antiviral drugs, vitamins, corticosteroids, anticoagulants, and antibiotics based on the condition of the child [13]. Recently, the US Food and Drug Administration (FDA) has approved the use of the Pfizer-BioNTech COVID-19 vaccine in children aged 12 years, and older, and children between 5 and 11 years are also covered for the prevention of COVID-19 [14].

2. Comparison between the prevalence of COVID-19 disease in South African children and children from other countries

COVID-19 is reported to have been transmitted by the intermediate host pangolin to an adult human being in China and the rest of the world and South Africa [7–9, 15]. COVID-19 in children is mainly transmitted through contact with those infected with SARS-CoV-2 (**Figure 1**) and the period of virus incubation is from 24 hours to 14 days [13, 16]. The virus spreads through contact with respiratory droplets, and COVID-19 in most children can also be excreted through urine, feces, aerosols, and body fluids that also contaminate the environment and continue the circle of infection (**Figure 1**) [13]. Children with COVID-19 have milder symptoms affecting the respiratory, gastrointestinal tract, and neurological systems [13, 16]. COVID-19 symptoms and signs in children

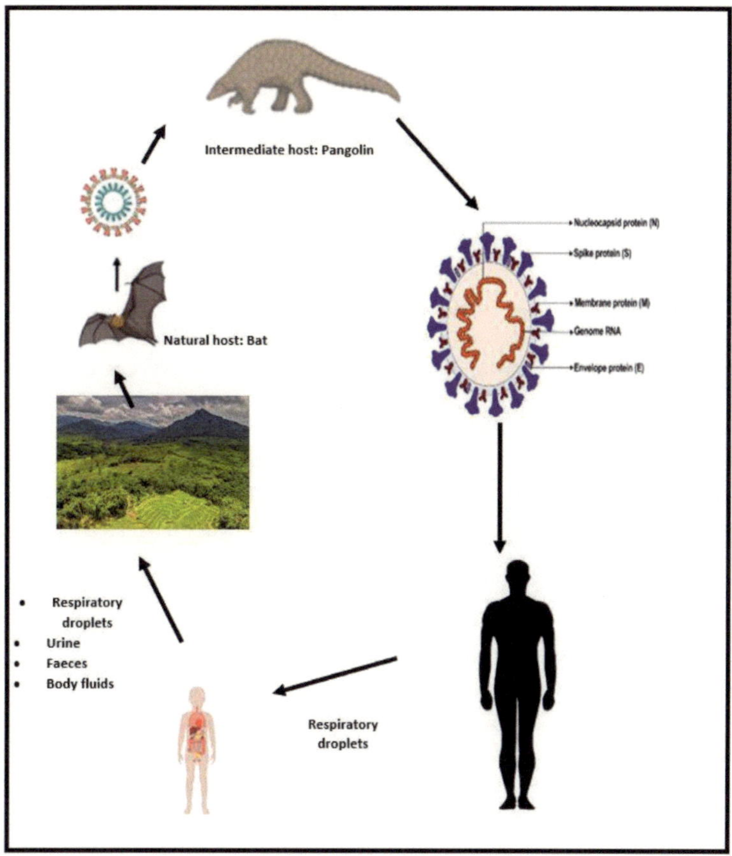

Figure 1.
SARS-CoV-2 transmission from the environment, animals, humans, and children.

include fever, cough, nasal congestion, headache, dyspnea, sore throat, ageusia, anosmia, abdominal pain, diarrhea, nausea, vomiting, lack of appetite, malaise, and myalgia [17]. Other children can become critically ill, and require hospitalization, intensive care, or mechanical ventilation or die, or in rare cases develop multisystem inflammatory syndrome (MIS) [13, 15, 16]. MIS is characterized by hypotension, pulmonary edema, and edema of other organs, necessitating intensive care to support the heart and lungs [16]. The first case of MIS-C in SA was reported in August 2020 in Cape Town [17]. COVID-19 is more prevalent in adults than in children less than 18 years [11, 16, 18].

2.1 Worldwide distribution and SA

There is still the continuation of the COVID-19 pandemic in Africa and globally [9]. WHO global COVID-19 reports on January 06, 2023 indicated that there are 657,977,736 cases of morbidity and 6,681,433 cases of mortality, and Europe has the highest number of confirmed cases of COVID-19, whereas Africa has the lowest cases [18]. The first positive case of COVID-19 in the African continent was confirmed on February 14, 2020 in Egypt, followed by Nigeria on February 28, 2020, and in SA on March 5, 2020 [5, 9]. There are currently 9,453,366 confirmed cases of COVID-19, 4,049,319 cases of morbidity, and 102,568 cases of mortality in SA as on January 06, 2023 [19, 20].

2.2 COVID-19 distribution in SA children and children from other countries 2020-2023

The prevalence of COVID-19 in children is lower than in adults worldwide [13, 21–24]. However, severe cases of morbidity and mortality have occurred in children [23]. In comparison to adults, there are few studies on COVID-19 in children [25]. There are gaps in the knowledge of the epidemiology of COVID-19 among children and adolescents worldwide [26]. In SA, on September 2020, the total laboratory-confirmed COVID-19 cases in South African children were 228 per 100,000 and were lower than the 829 per 100,000 children in the United States. COVID-19 cases in children in SA were higher compared to rates of less than 100 per 100,000 children in Norway and Australia [10]. UNICEF report from 96 countries in 2020 has indicated that children and adolescents less than 20 years have accounted for 21% of the COVID-19 cases and 33% of the 2020 population [27]. According to the UNICEF data, at the beginning of January 2023, there were 4,400,000 mortality reports globally. From those reports, 17,200 deaths occurred in children and adolescents less than 20 years, and 53% of those cases occurred in adolescents aged 10 to 19 years, whereas 47% of the cases occurred among children aged 0 to 9 years [28].

3. Risk factors predisposing South African children to COVID-19 disease compared to other countries

There are few studies conducted on the epidemiology and clinical manifestation of COVID-19 in African children in comparison to continents such as China, Europe, and North America [10, 21, 29]. The findings of studies from other countries cannot be generalizable to South African children because of the differences in the risk factors predisposing children to COVID-19, mostly the burden of infectious diseases [10]. SA children are affected by HIV, TB, malnutrition, childhood obesity, overcrowding, chronic kidney disease, malignancy, heart conditions, asthma, diabetes, and limited access to quality health care [10]. However, the study conducted in six African countries namely SA, Congo, Ghana, Kenya, Nigeria, and Uganda from March 01, 2020, to December 31, 2020 on COVID-19 children and adolescents has revealed the highest mortality and morbidity rates due to comorbidity with non-infectious diseases [21]. In the United States, and North America, important risk factors in children include hypertension, obesity, neuropsychiatric disorders, cardiac or circulatory anomalies, chronic lung disease, and immunosuppression [21, 22]. In China, children are at risk of developing severe COVID-19 cases due to underlying

	SA	China	North America
Risk factors	HIV, TB, malnutrition, childhood obesity, overcrowding, limited access to quality healthcare, diabetes, asthma, heart conditions, malignancy, chronic, kidney disease, and hypertension [10, 30, 31]	Circulatory or cardiac congenital anomalies, obesity, essential hypertension, epilepsy, malnutrition, asthma, Down syndrome, neuropsychiatric disorders, leukemia, hydronephrosis, and intussusception [13, 22].	Hypertension, obesity, diabetes, neuropsychiatric disorders, cardiac, or circulatory anomalies [21]

Table 1.
Comparison of the risk factors predisposing South African children to COVID-19 in comparison to other countries.

conditions such as circulatory or heart congenital anomalies, obesity, essential hypertension, epilepsy, malnutrition, asthma, Down syndrome, neuropsychiatric disorders, hydronephrosis, leukemia, and intussusception (**Table 1**) [13, 22].

4. Diagnosis, prevention, and treatment of COVID-19 disease in children in South Africa and other countries

4.1 Diagnosis of COVID-19 disease in children in South Africa and other countries

COVID-19 diagnosis is defined based on clinical manifestations, laboratory testing, and chest radiograph imaging, including asymptomatic infection, as mild, moderate, severe, or critical [24]. According to WHO, clinical diagnosis depends on disease severity, where (1) non-severe indicates the absence of signs of severe or critical disease, and (2) severe by oxygen saturation less than 90% on room air, signs of pneumonia, or respiratory distress, and (3) critical, the patients require treatment and presents with acute respiratory distress, sepsis, or shock [32]. The laboratory diagnosis of COVID-19 in SA (**Table 2**) is by using the SARS-CoV-2 reverse-transcription real-time polymerase chain reaction (rRT-PCR) on a respiratory sample obtained from a nasopharyngeal or oropharyngeal swab and SARS-CoV-2 antigen-based testing [10, 11, 30]. In other

Continent/Country	Diagnosis Laboratory diagnosis
1. SA	rRT-PCR, SARS-CoV-2 antigen-based test [10, 11, 33]
2. China	RT-PCR, viral antigen test, and serology test [12, 16, 23, 32]
3. America	RT-PCR, viral antigen test, and serology test [12, 16, 23, 32]
Continent/Country	**Prevention COVID-19 Vaccines**
1. SA	Pfizer-BioNTech, BNT162b2 [11, 14, 34]
2. China	BNT162b2 [34]
3. America	Pfizer-BioNTech, BNT162b2, Sinovac [14, 25, 26, 34]
4. Argentina	BNT162b2, Sinopharm [34, 35]
5. Colombia	AstraZeneca, Moderna, Sinopharm, Johnson, and Johnson [35]
6. El Salvador	Sinovac [35]
7. Ecuador	Sinovac [35]
8. Brazil	BNT162b2 [34]
9. Finland	BNT162b2 [34]
10. Poland	BNT162b2 [34]
11. Turkey	BNT162b2 [34]
12. Spain	BNT162b2 [34]
13. Germany	BNT162b2 [34]
14. Europe	Spikevax [34]

Table 2.
Diagnosis and prevention of COVID-19 for South African children and adolescents versus children and adolescents from other countries/continents.

places such as China and the American continent, laboratory diagnosis (**Table 2**) is by reverse transcription-polymerase chain reaction (RT-PCR) of nasopharyngeal and oropharyngeal swabs, viral antigen, and serology test [12, 16, 23, 33].

4.2 Prevention of COVID-19 disease in children in South Africa and other countries

The worldwide COVID-19 vaccine nation strategies had initially focused mainly on adults because children were less affected [14]. However, the emergence of mutations in the SARS-CoV-2 genome such as delta and omicron variants increased the risk of infections in children and adolescents in various countries [11, 14]. In SA, various variants emerged during the first and fourth waves of the COVID-19 epidemic; the Wuhan-Hu in the first wave between weeks 24 and 34 of 2020, the Beta variant during the second wave between week 47 of 2020 and week 5 of 2021 [11, 36]. The Delta variant caused the third wave between weeks 19 and 37 of 2021, and the omicron variant was responsible for the fourth wave between week 48 of 2021 and week 5 of 2022. Currently, several countries have approved the use of COVID-19 vaccines in children and adolescents (**Table 2**) [14]. The FDA has approved the use of the Pfizer-BioNTech COVID-19 vaccine in children aged 5 to 12 years [14, 25, 26]. Furthermore, SA approved the use of the Pfizer-BioNTech COVID-19 vaccine in children aged 12–17 years on October 20, 2021 (**Table 2**) [11, 14]. The Spikevax vaccine is approved by the European Medicines Agency to be used in adolescents aged 12 to 17 years (**Table 2**) [34]. FDA has authorized the emergency use of the BNT162b2 vaccine in children and adolescents aged 12 years and above in countries including, the United States, China, Finland, Spain, Turkey, Poland, Germany, Brazil, Argentina, and SA (**Table 2**) [34]. Other licensed vaccines for children and adolescents in Latin America include the Sinovac COVID-19 vaccine in Chile for children over 6 years, and in El Salvador for children aged 6 to 11 years, the Sinovac COVID-19 vaccine (**Table 2**) [35]. Sinopharm COVID-19 vaccine is licensed in Argentina for children as young as three years old and the Sinovac vaccine is used in Ecuador for children from six years old (**Table 2**) [35]. COVID-19 vaccines from AstraZeneca, Moderna, Sinopharm,

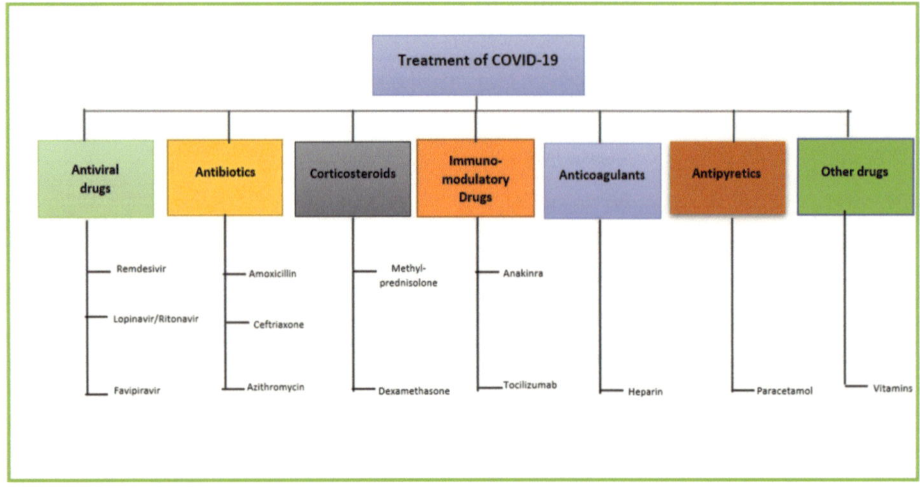

Figure 2.
Drugs used in the treatment of COVID-19 in adults and children worldwide.

and Johnson and Johnson are used in Colombia for children 12 years and older, and vaccination in Costa Rica is from 12 years (**Table 2**) [35].

4.3 Treatment of COVID-19 disease in children in South Africa and other countries

The treatment of COVID-19 is still evolving, and the clinical trials are ongoing, and the current recommendations depend on previous experiments and clinical trials [31]. Moreover, pharmacological management in children and adolescents is extrapolated from adult studies [31]. Management of COVID-19 is based on categories including (1) no treatment for asymptomatic cases, (2) antipyretic therapy in moderate and mild cases, and (3) for critical cases several drugs [37]. COVID-19 pharmacological management in children includes antiviral drugs (remdesivir, lopinavir/ritonavir, and favipiravir), antibiotics (amoxicillin, ceftriaxone, and azithromycin), vitamins, corticosteroids (methylprednisolone and dexamethasone), immunomodulatory drugs (anakinra and tocilizumab), anticoagulant (heparin), antipyretic drug (paracetamol), and hydroxychloroquine, based on the condition of the child (**Figure 2**) [13, 37].

5. Conclusions

The current review documents the prevalence, risk factors, and management of COVID-19 disease in South African children and adolescents in comparison to other countries in other continents. There is limited literature, and few studies covering the epidemiology of COVID-19 in SA and other countries in Africa and other continents. COVID-19 is less prevalent in children across the countries covered in this review when compared to adults. The burden of COVID-19 is higher in children in countries like the United States when compared to SA. There are similarities in the risk factors which predispose South African children to COVID-19 and children in other countries, except that the burden of bacterial and viral infection is higher in Africa and SA. Moreover, living conditions, poverty, and quality and access to healthcare facilities are still a challenge in SA and other African countries. Clinical and laboratory diagnosis is similar and laboratory diagnosis in SA and other countries is mainly through rRT-PCR, RT-PCR, SARS-CoV-2 viral antigen, and serology tests. Various vaccines including Pfizer-BioNTech COVID-19 vaccine, Spikevax, BNT162b2, AstraZeneca, Moderna, Sinopharm, and Johnson and Johnson are approved and licensed for use in children and adolescents in various countries including SA. There are limited studies defining country-based pharmacological management of COVID-19 in children.

Acknowledgements

We acknowledge Walter Sisulu University, Department of Internal Medicine and Pharmacology, and the Central University of Technology, Department of Health Sciences, and National Research Foundation.

Conflict of interest

The authors declare no conflict of interest.

Author details

Moleboheng Emily Binyane[1] and Polo-Ma-Abiele Hildah Mfengwana[2*]

1 Department of Internal Medicine and Pharmacology, Walter Sisulu University, Mthatha, South Africa

2 Department of Health Sciences, Central University of Technology, Bloemfontein, South Africa

*Address all correspondence to: pntsoeli@cut.ac.za

References

[1] Cascella M, Rajnik M, Cuomo A, Dulebohn SC, Di Napoli R. Features, Evaluation and Treatment Coronavirus (COVID-19). StatPearls: NCBI Bookshelf; 2020. pp. 1-17. Available from: https://www.ncbi.nlm.nih.gov/books/NBK554776/?report= print able [Accessed: April 1, 2023]

[2] Baker RE, Mahmud AS, Miller IF, Rajeev M, Rasambainarivo F, Rice BL, et al. Reviews infectious disease in an era of global change. Nature Reviews Microbiology. 2022;**20**:193-205. DOI: 10.1038/s41579-021-00639-z

[3] Nicola M, Alsafi Z, Sohrabic C, Kerwand A, Al-Jabird A, Iosifidisc C, et al. The socio-economic implications of the coronavirus pandemic (COVID-19): A review. International Journal of Surgery. 2020;**78**:185-193. DOI: 10.1016/j.ijsu.2020.04.018

[4] Binyane ME, Mfengwana PH. Traditional medicinal plants as the potential adjuvant, prophylactic and treatment therapy for Covid-19 disease: A review. IntechOpen. 2022:**4**:53-73. DOI: 10.5772/intechopen.104491

[5] Lone SA, Ahmad A. COVID-19 pandemic–an African perspective. Emerging Microbes and Infections. 2020;**9**:1300-1308. DOI:10.1080/22221751.2020.1775132

[6] Chali BU, Melaku T, Berhanu N, Mengistu B, Milkessa G, Mamo G, et al. Traditional medicine practice in the context of COVID-19 pandemic: Community claim in Jimma zone, Oromia. Ethiopia. Infection and Drug Resistance. 2021;**14**:3773-3783. DOI: 10.2147/IDR.S331434

[7] Singla R, Mishra A, Joshi R, Jha S, Sharma AR, Upadhyay S, et al. Human animal interface of SARS-CoV-2 (COVID-19) transmission: A critical appraisal of scientific evidence. Veterinary Research Communications. 2020;**44**:119-130. DOI: 10.1007/s11259-020-09781-0

[8] Mahdy MAA, Younis W, Ewaida Z. An overview of SARS-CoV-2 and animal infection. Frontiers in Veterinary Science. 2020;**7**(596391):1-12. DOI: 10.3389/fvets.2020.596391

[9] Giandhari J, Pillay S, Wilkinson E, Tegally H, Sinayskiy I, Schuld M, et al. Early transmission of SARS-CoV-2 in South Africa: An epidemiological and phylogenetic report. PubMed Central. 2020;**2020**:1-17. DOI: 10.1101/2020.05.29.20116376

[10] Kufa T, Jassat W, Cohen C, Tempia S, Masha M, Wolter N, et al. Epidemiology of SARS-CoV-2 infection and SARS-CoV-2 positive hospital admissions among children in South Africa. Wiley. 2021;**16**(1):34-47. DOI: 10.1111/irv.12916

[11] Chiwandire N, Jassat W, Groome M, Kufa T, Walaza S, Wolter N, et al. Changing epidemiology of COVID-19 in children and adolescents over four successive epidemic waves in South Africa, 2020-2022. The Lancet. 2022;**2022**:1-25. DOI: 10.2139/ssrn.4169800

[12] Su L, Ma X, Yu H, Zhang Z, Bian P, Han Y, et al. The different clinical characteristics of corona virus disease cases between children and their families in China – The character of children with COVID-19. Emerging Microbes and Infections. 2020;**9**(1):707-713. DOI: 10.1080/22221751.2020.1744 483

[13] Wang L, Li G, Yuan C, Yang Y, Ling G, Zheng J, et al. Progress in the

diagnosis and treatment of COVID-19 in children: A review. International Journal of General Medicine. 2021;**14**:8097-8108. DOI: 10.2147/IJGM. S335888

[14] Govender K, Nyamaruze P, McKerrowN, Meyer-WeitzA, CowdenRG. COVID-19 vaccines for children and adolescents in Africa: Aligning our priorities to situational realities. BMJ Global Health. 2022;7(e007839):1-8. DOI: 10.1136/bmjgh-2021-007839

[15] Wiersinga WJ, Rhodes A, Cheng AC, Peacock SJ, Prescott HC. Pathophysiology, transmission, diagnosis, and treatment of coronavirus disease 2019 (COVID-19) a review. Journal of the American Medical Association. 2020;**324**(8):782-793. DOI: 10.1001/jama.2020.12839

[16] Melo MM, Neta MMR, Neto ARS, Carvalho ARB, Magalhães RLB, Valle ARMC, et al. Symptoms of COVID-19 in children. Brazilian Journal of Medical and Biological Research. 2022;**55**(e12038):1-7. DOI: 10.1590/1414-431X2022e12038

[17] Saggers RT. COVID-19 and multi-system inflammatory syndrome in children. Wits Journal of Clinical Medicine. 2021;**3**(1):43-48. DOI: 10.18772/26180197.2021 v3n1a6

[18] Pierce CA, Herold KC, Herold BC, Chou J, Randolph A, Kane B, et al. COVID-19 and children. Science. 2022;**377**(6611):1144-1149. DOI: 10.1126/science.ade1675

[19] World Health Organisation (WHO). Health Emergency Dashboard (COVID-19). Available from: https://covid19.who.int/. [Accessed: August 01, 2023]

[20] Johns Hopkins University Center for Systems Science and Engineering (JHU CSSE). COVID-19 Dashboard statistics new cases and deaths South Africa. Available from: https://www.google.com/search?sxsrf=AJOqlzXJEr5sXlbv6bfMLSCG8ZsXS_cYfQ:1673188761516&q=COVID19&si=AEcPFx7eHRJU0tWbjC5cc2C2rVygfPuoetC2JDc0IDqLp89f-Ps4nHnOQ1RU8-xfCXL9ib2X30cyRoVTgouLhPG0LpiFNLabOH5KOFW4oJ7q50YOdrNFuM%3D&biw=1366&bih=657&dpr=1. [Accessed: August 01, 2023]

[21] Sam-Agudu NA, Rabie H, Pipo MT, Byamungu LN, Masekela R, van der Zalm MM, et al. The critical need for pooled data on coronavirus disease 2019 in African children: An AFREhealth call for action through multicountry research collaboration. Clinical Infectious Diseases. 2021;**73**(10):1913-1919. DOI: 10.1093/cid/ciab142

[22] Nachega JB, Sam-Agudu NA, Machekano RN, Rabie H, van der Zalm MM, Redfern A, et al. Assessment of clinical outcomes among children and adolescents hospitalized with COVID-19 in 6 Sub-Saharan African countries. Journal of American Medical Association Paediatrics. 2022;**176**(3):e216436. DOI: 10.1001/jamapediatrics.2021.6436

[23] Tsabouri S, Makis A, Kosmeri C, Siomou E. Risk factors for severity in children with coronavirus disease 2019. Pediatric Clinics of North America. 2021;**68**(1):321-338. DOI: 10.1016/j.pcl.2020.07.014

[24] Woodruff RC, Campbell AP, Taylor CA, Chai SJ, Kawasaki B, Meek J, et al. Risk factors for severe COVID-19 in children. Pediatrics. 2022;**149**(1):e20210534. DOI: 10.1542/peds.2021-053418

[25] Dong Y, Mo X, Hu Y, Qi X, Jiang F, Jiang Z, et al. Epidemiology of COVID-19 among children in China.

Pediatrics. 2020;**145**(6):1-12. DOI: 10.1542/peds.2020-0702

[26] Guo C-X, He L, Yin J-Y, Meng X-G, Tan W, Yang G-P, et al. Epidemiological and clinical features of paediatric COVID-19. BMC Medicine. 2020;**18**(250):1, 250-7. DOI: 10.1186/s12916-020-01719-22020

[27] Unicef data. COVID-19 confirmed cases and deaths age and sex-disaggregated data [Accessed: January 17, 2023]

[28] Unicef data. Child mortality and COVID-19. Available from: https://seotest.buzz/topic/child-survival/covid-19/. [Accessed: January 17, 2023]

[29] Coker M, Folayan MO, Michelow IC, Oladokun RE, Torbunde N, Agudu NA. Things must not fall apart: The ripple effects of the COVID-19 pandemic on children in sub-Saharan Africa. Pediatric Research. 2021;**89**:1078-1086. DOI: 10.1038/s41390-020-01174-y

[30] Brooke B, Frean J, Blumberg L, Cohen C, Govender N, Ismail N, et al. Epidemiology and clinical characteristics of laboratory confirmed COVID-19 among children and adolescents aged ≤18 years, South Africa, 1 March –19 September 2020. The National Institute for Communicable Diseases 2020;**2020**:1-14. Available from: https://www.nicd.ac.za/wp-content/uploads /2020/10/Monthly-Covid-19-In-Children-Surveillance-Report-2.pdf. [Accessed: November 1, 2023]

[31] Parasher A. COVID-19: Current understanding of its pathophysiology, clinical presentation and treatment. Postgraduate Medical Journal. 2021;**97**(1147):312-320. DOI: 10.1136/postgradmedj-2020-138577

[32] World Health Organization (WHO). Clinical management of COVID-19. 2023:1-182. Available from: file:///C:/Users/moleb/Downloads/WHO-2019-nCoV-clinical-2023.1-eng%20(2).pdf. [Accessed: January 21, 2023]

[33] Yousaf AR, Cortese MM, Taylor AW, Broder R, Joshua M, Wong JM, et al. Reported cases of multisystem inflammatory syndrome in children aged 12-20 years in the USA who received a COVID-19 vaccine, December, 2020, Through August, 2021: A surveillance investigation. Lancet Child Adolescent Health. **2022**(6):303-312. DOI: 10.1016/S2352-4642(22)00028-1

[34] Lv M, Luo X, Shen Q, Lei R, Liu X, Liu E, et al. Safety, immunogenicity, and efficacy of COVID-19 vaccines in children and adolescents: A systematic review. Vaccine. 2021;**9**(10):1102-1114. DOI: 10.3390/vaccines9101102

[35] Rodriguez-Morales AJ, León-Figueroa DA, Romaní L, Mchugh TD, Leblebicioglu H. Vaccination of children against COVID-19: The experience in Latin America. Annals of Clinical Microbiology and Antimicrobials. 2022;**21**(14):1-5. DOI: 10.1186/s12941-022-00505-7

[36] Mwangi P, Okendo J, Mogotsi M, Ogunbayo A, Adelabu O, Sondlane H, et al. SARS-CoV2 variants from COVID-19 positive cases in the Free State Province, South Africa from July 2020 to December 2021. Frontiers in Virology. 2020;**2**:935. DOI: 10.3389/fviro.2022.935131

[37] Venturini E, Montagnani C, Garazzino S, Donà D, Pierantoni L, Lo Vecchio A, et al. Treatment of children with COVID-19: Position paper of the Italian Society of Pediatric Infectious Disease. Italian Journal of Pediatrics. 2022;**46**(139):1-11. DOI: 10.1186/s/3052-020-00900-w

Chapter 4

Epidemiology of SARS-CoV-2 Infection in Mexico and Latin America

Nicolás Padilla-Raygoza, Gilberto Flores-Vargas, María de Jesús Gallardo-Luna, Efraín Navarro-Olivos, Guadalupe Irazú Morales-Reyes and Jessica Paola Plascencia-Roldán

Abstract

This chapter presents some insights into COVID-19 in children. We begin by summarizing the fundamental aspects of SARS-CoV-2 and COVID-19. We also cover issues about the severity of the disease and fatality and factors associated with the outcome of pediatric patients with COVID-19. Most evidence treated in this chapter comes from reports in Mexico, but a general landscape in Latin America is pictured. COVID-19 does not seem to be so severe among children. It is worth noting that those at higher risk are the children between 0 and 2 years who develop pneumonia. In this chapter, we did not discuss extensively the Multisystem Inflammatory Syndrome nor the social impact that the COVID-19 pandemic has had on children. Many studies used for this chapter relied on open data sources resulting from a surveillance system designed for the general population. Therefore, specific variables for children were not analyzed.

Keywords: COVID-19, SARS-CoV-2, children, pneumonia, epidemiology, fatality

1. Introduction

In November-December 2019, several cases of pneumonia of an unknown origin were reported in Wuhan, China, and the World Health Organization (WHO) declared a public health emergency of international concern [1].

From then until October 2022, the outbreak spread to 237 countries, with 626,565,321 confirmed cases, of which 6,566,037 died [2].

The Pan American Health Organization (PAHO) [3] reported on November 5, 2022, the confirmed cases, of all ages, in the Americas region (**Table 1**).

In Mexico, until 31 October, 2022, 7,111,119 confirmed cases had been reported, and from them, 330,393 had been reported dead, with a Case Fatality Ratio (CFR) of 4.65% [2].

Region	Confirmed cases	Deaths	Case Fatality Ratio
North America	107,924,403	1,439,525	1.33
Central America	4013, 243	53,616	13.30
South America	64,184,548	1,329,987	0.20
Caribbean and Atlantic Ocean Islands	4,239,152	35,327	0.83
Null	10,869,300	219,088	2.02
Total	191,230,646	3,077,543	1.61

Source: Pan American Health Organization [3].

Table 1.
Distribution of confirmed cases, deaths, and Case Fatality Ratio for COVID-19 by area of America.

Since the beginning of the pandemic, it was reported that the highest frequency of cases and case fatalities were in men aged 45 years and older [4]. The affectation in children under 18 years of age was lower than in the general population, and the form of COVID-19 was less severe [5].

In China, Dong et al. [5] reported 728 confirmed cases, mostly men, with a median of 7 years. Approximately 90% of the cases were asymptomatic, mild, or moderate.

2. SARS-CoV-2

Two new coronaviruses emerged and induced severe illnesses during the last 20 years. One of them is the severe respiratory syndrome coronavirus (SARS-CoV-1). It appeared in 2002 in Guangdong, China, and spread to 29 countries, with 8098 confirmed cases and 774 deaths, with a CFR of 9.6% [6, 7], and 135 reported pediatric cases (1.7% of cases) with no deaths [8].

In 2012, Middle East Respiratory Syndrome Coronavirus (MERS-CoV) emerged in Saudi Arabia, resulting in 2494 cases with 858 deaths in 27 countries, with a CFR of 34.4% [9].

Coronaviruses belong to the Coronaviridae family in the Nidovirales order [10]. In nature, four coronavirus subfamilies have been identified: alpha, beta, gamma, and delta. Alpha and beta coronaviruses apparently develop in mammals—specifically in bats—while gamma and delta have been found in pigs and poultry [10]. Corona represents the crown-like spikes on the outer surface of the virus; thus, it was named a coronavirus, which is small (65—125 nm in diameter) and contains a genome (RNA) that varies between 26 kb and 32 kb [11].

The SARS-CoV-2 was identified and characterized by Zhu et al. [12]. It uses the same cell entry receptor—Angiotensin-Converting Enzyme.

2 (ACE-2)—as SARS-CoV, highly expressed in airway epithelial cells and in other organism cells [8]. Also, Zhu et al. [8] reported the cytopathic effects and morphology. It is a member of a family of coronaviruses that infect humans. This virus grows more in human airway epithelial cells than tissue culture cells, suggesting the potential for increased infectivity in the respiratory tract.

The glycosylated spike (S) protein of SARS-CoV-2 has a 10-fold greater affinity to bind to ACE-2 than SARS-CoV-1 [13, 14].

Initially, transmission occurred from an intermediate zoonotic host to humans and later by effective human-to-human [15]. The primary transmission route is through respiratory droplets when a sick person coughs, sneezes, or speaks [16].

There are no reports of transmission of the infection through transfusions or organ transplants [17].

3. Coronavirus disease (COVID-19)

Cui et al. [18] reported in a meta-analysis that 17% of COVID-19 cases were in children less than 1 year, 24% between 1 and 5 years, 20% between 6 and 10 years, 20% between 11 and 15 years, and 18% from 15 or more years. 55% of the sample was male. Regarding the severity of COVID-19, 20% were asymptomatic, 33% mild, 51% moderate, and 7% severe, and they did not report any deaths [18]. **Table 2** shows the predominant clinical data according to Cui et al. [18].

Dyspnea has been reported in 13% of the cases [19], and other reports have mentioned headaches and chills (both in approximately 28%) [8].

Not testing widely in many countries made it difficult to quantify the burden of SARS-CoV-2 infection in children [17].

In Mexico, the subjects who meet an operational definition undergo a COVID-19 test (RT-PCR or antigen detection). A suspected case of viral respiratory disease is anyone with cough, fever, dyspnea (severe), or headache, having at least one of the following: myalgias, arthralgias, odynophagia, chills, chest pain, rhinorrhea, anosmia, dysgeusia, or conjunctivitis. In children under five years, irritability is interchangeable with headache [20, 21].

Clinical data	%	CI95%
Fever	51	45–57
Cough	41	35–47
Sore throat	16	7–25
Tachycardia	12	3–21
Rhinorrhea	14	8–19
Nasal congestion	17	6–27
Tachypnea	9	4–14
Diarrhea	8	6–11
Vomiting	7	5–10
Myalgia or fatigue	12	7–17
Hypoxemia	3	1–4
Chest pain	3	0–5

CI95% Confidence Interval 95%.
Source: Cui et al. [18].

Table 2.
Distribution of clinical data in children under 18 years old.

4. COVID-19 severity

One limitation in Mexico and other countries was that RT-PCR was performed only for symptomatic patients. It led to underestimating the burden of the pandemic and underreporting of children with mild or asymptomatic COVID-19 [17]. In a joint WHO-China work, it was reported that of 55,924 confirmed cases, 2.4% were in children under 19 years of age, and of them, 2.5% developed severe disease and 0.2% critical illness [22].

In China, when studying 728 pediatric patients with confirmed COVID-19, 12.9% presented asymptomatic symptoms, 43.1% mild, 40.9% moderate, 2.5% severe, and 0.4% critical [5]. In Italy, 1.2% of the COVID-19 cases were in children under 18 years of age, and no deaths were reported [23]. In the USA, 1.7% of the cases were in children under 18 years of age [19]. In Spain, only 0.8% of the cases were in children under 18 years of age [24].

Multisystem Inflammatory Syndrome (MIS-C) was reported as related to COVID-19 and is associated with Unit Intensive Care admissions and death [25, 26]. In Latin American children, the age where the MIS-C occurred most frequently was over 10 years (35.8%) [27].

There are features in common between MIS-C and Kawasaki disease [28]. In Europe, a thirty-fold increase in the incidence of Kawasaki disease has been reported [25]. Nevertheless, a more severe Kawasaki disease was reported in children older than 5 years and was called atypical Kawasaki disease [29]. In Latin America, up to August 2020, 95 cases of MIS-C in children were reported; 54.7% were men, 11 had a pre-existing medical condition before MIS-C, 21% were admitted to intensive care, and two died [27].

5. Pneumonia

Pneumonia is considered a leading cause of death in COVID-19 patients of any age.

The development of pneumonia was the chief risk factor for mortality, with a risk of 6.45%. For those who required intubation, it increased to 8.75% [30].

In Mexico, up to May 2020, of 1443 children with COVID-19, 9.8% had pneumonia [30]. Among 141 children with pneumonia and COVID-19, the higher effect was in children under 1 year (OR = 5.83 CI95% 3.56–9.54). The male sex manifested itself as a weak protective factor for developing pneumonia (OR = 0.73 CI95% 0.51–1.04); diabetes showed a strong effect (OR = 12.61 CI95% 4.62–34.41), and the same happened with immunosuppression (OR = 7.35 CI95% 3.97–13.61) [31]. Antúnez-Montes et al. [27] also found a statistically significant relation between pneumonia and pediatric ICU admission.

6. Fatality of cases

In Mexico, until May 2020, the CFR was 0.23% for those between 0 and 5 years and 0.06% for those between 6 and 11 years [32].

Navarro et al. [33] reported that of 48,505 confirmed cases up to December 31, 2020, the CFR was the highest for children between 0 and 2 years of age (3.99), the highest among the Mexican child population. For pneumonia, the CFR was 15.46%,

Country	Confirmed cases in less than 19 years old		Deaths in less than 19 years old	
	n	%	n	%
Argentina	1003	1.2	0	0.00
Bolivia	446	11.6	ND	ND
Brazil	4019	3.4	94	0.24
Chile	4348	9.4	0	0.00
Colombia	2087	11.8	6	0.95
Costa Rica	55	6.1	0	0.00
Cuba	238	12.5	0	0.00
Ecuador	490	1.4	6	0.21
El Salvador	102	6.4	1	3.13
Guatemala	278	12.2	ND	ND
Haiti	44	7.3	2	9.09
Honduras	204	7.2	0	0.00
Mexico	1376	2.4	9	0.15
Panama	830	8.4	ND	ND
Paraguay	184	22.0	ND	ND
Peru	4350	4.7	17	0.64
Dominican Republic	544	5.9	4	1.51
Uruguay	14	1.9	ND	ND
Venezuela	145	17.5	ND	ND

Source: Taken and modified from [34].

Table 3.
Distribution of confirmed cases of COVID-19 and deaths from this cause in Latin American countries.

but the OR was 63.90%, showing the strong effect of pneumonia on mortality in Mexican children.

Confirmed cases of SARS-CoV-2 infection and deaths, in Latin America, in children under 19 years are reported in **Table 3**, up to May 2020.

Case fatality ranged from 0 to 9.09%. The countries with recorded deaths were Brazil, Colombia, Ecuador, El Salvador, Haiti, Mexico, Peru, and the Dominican Republic. These cases might have had some underlying comorbidity. For children, mortality is infrequent, and those admitted to intensive care units usually have a chronic or preexisting condition [27, 34].

As reported, case fatality is lower among children (0.39%) than in later ages (99.61%) [35].

7. Sex

In a report from China of SARS-CoV-2 infection confirmed cases, men predominated with 57.4% [5]. Among 50 children from India with co-signed SARS-CoV-2, 64% were males [36].

Up to May 2020, in Mexico, 48% of the children with COVID-19 were males, and 44.4% of those who died were men [30]. Moreno-Noguez M et al. [31] report similar results on close dates.

In Mexico, until December 31, 2020, among 48,505 confirmed cases of COVID-19, males (50.43%) and females (49.57%), the CFR was 96% for males and 0.80% for females under 18 years of age [33].

It is important to note that these reports are from the same public database of the Mexican government at different times, and there is not much difference in the results.

8. Age

Dong et al. [5] reported that among 728 confirmed cases of infection by SARS-CoV-2, 24.7% were 11—15 years old, followed by 6—10 years old (23.4%).

In Mexico, the CFR was 3.99% in children under 2 years and 0.45% in those between 12 and 17 years of age [33].

9. Comorbidities

Navarro et al. [33] report that comorbidities representing a risk of dying in adults do not have this role in the pediatric population. Tsankov et al. [37] report in a meta-analysis that comorbidities increase the risk of severe COVID-19 and mortality in children. Nevertheless, studies in the meta-analysis only included one Latin American population.

10. Conclusions

SARS-CoV-2 is a coronavirus that emerged in late 2019. Its associated disease, COVID-19, spread to almost all the world. COVID-19 seems to be mild in children. Up to May 2020, infections by SARS-CoV-2 were scarce among children in Latin America, and so were the deaths by COVID-19. The children at higher risk are those between 0 and 2 years. Most deaths were among the ones with pneumonia. Comorbidities commonly associated with poor outcomes in adults did not play a crucial role in children. The societal impact of COVID-19 on children was not treated in this chapter.

Conflict of interest

The authors declare no conflict of interest.

Author details

Nicolás Padilla-Raygoza[1*], Gilberto Flores-Vargas[1],
María de Jesús Gallardo-Luna[1], Efraín Navarro-Olivos[2],
Guadalupe Irazú Morales-Reyes[1] and Jessica Paola Plascencia-Roldán[1]

1 Department of Research and Technological Development, Directorate of Teaching and Research, Institute of Public Health from Guanajuato State, Mexico

2 Directorate of Teaching and Research, Institute of Public Health from Guanajuato State, Mexico

*Address all correspondence to: npadillar@guanajuato.gob.mx

References

[1] World Health Organization. Rolling updates on coronavirus disease (COVID-19); 2020. Available from: https://www.who.int/emergencies/diseases/novel-coronavirus-2019/events-as-they-happen. [Accessed: November 7, 2022]

[2] Subsecretaría de Prevención y Promoción de la Salud. Informe técnico semanal COVID-19 México. 1 noviembre 2022. Disponible en: https://www.gob.mx/salud/documentos/informe-tecnico-diario-covid19-2022?idiom=es. [Accessed: November 11, 2022]

[3] Health Organization. Cumulative confirmed and probable COVID-19 cases reported by Countries and Territories in the región of the Americas. 2022. Available from: https://ais.paho.org/phip/viz/COVID19Table.asp. [Accessed: November 12, 2022]

[4] Padilla-Raygoza N, Flores-Vargas G, Navarro-Olivos E, Lara-Lona E, Gallardo-Luna MJ, Magos-Vázquez FJ, et al. Relationship of clinical data and confirmed case of disease by the new coronavirus, in the Mexican state of Guanajuato. Journal of Advances in Medicine and Medical Research. 2020;**32**(23):73-84. DOI: 10.9734/JAMMR/2020/v32i2330719

[5] Dong Y, Mo X, Hu Y, Qi X, Jiang F, Jiang Z, et al. Epidemiology of COVID-19 among children in China. Pediatrics. 2020;**145**(6):e20200702. DOI: 10.1542/peds.2020-0702

[6] World Health Organization. Summary of probable SARS cases with onset of illness from 1 November 202 to 31 2003. Geneva: WHO. Available from: https://www.who.int/csr/sars/country/table2004_04_21/en/. [Accessed November 15, 2022]

[7] Fung WK, Yu PLH. SARS case-fatality rates. CMAJ. 2003;**169**:277-278

[8] Stockman LJ, Massoudi MS, Helfand R, et al. Severe acute respiratory síndrome in children. The Pediatric Infectious Disease Journal. 2007;**26**:68-74. DOI: 10.1097/01.inf.0000247136.28950.41

[9] World Health Organization. Middle East Respiratory síndrome Coronavirus (MERS-CoV). Geneva: WHO. Available from: https://www.who.int/emergencies/mers-cov/en/. [Accessed: November 15, 2022]

[10] VelavanTP MCG. The COVID 19 epidemic. Tropical Medicine and International Health. 2020;**25**(3):278-280. DOI: 10.1111/tmi.13383

[11] Shereen MA, Khan S, Kazmi A, Bashir N, Siddiquea R. COVID-19 infection: Origin, transmission, and characteristics of human coronaviruses. Journal of Advanced Research. 2020;**24**:91-98. DOI: 10.1016/j.jare.2020.03.005

[12] Zhu N, Zhang D, Wang W, Li X, Yang B, Song J, et al. A novel coronavirus from patients with pneumonia in China, 2019. The New England Journal of Medicine. 2020;**382**(727):37. DOI: 10.1056/NEJMoa2

[13] Wilson ME, Chen LH. Travellers give wings to novel coronavirus (2019-nCoV). Journal of Travel Medicine. 2020;**27**:taaa15. DOI: 10.1093/jtm/taaa015

[14] Jin Y, Yang H, Ji W, et al. Virology epidemiology, pathogenesis, and control of COVID-19. Viruses. 2020;**12**:372. DOI: 10.3390/v12040372

[15] Zhou P, Yang X-L, Wang X-G, et al. A pneumonia outbreak associated with anew coronavirus of probable bat origin. Nature. 2020;**579**:270-273. DOI: 10.1038/s41586-020-2012-7

[16] Centers for Disease Control and Prevention. Coronavirus disease 2019 (COVID-19). 2020. Available from: https://www.cdc.gov/coronavirus/2019-ncov/need-extra-precautions/pregnancy-breastfeeding.html. [Accessed: November 17, 2022]

[17] Rajapakse N, Dixit D. Human and novel coronavirus infections in children: A review. Pediatrics and International Child Health. 2021;**41**(1):36-55. DOI: 10.1080/20469047.2020.1781356

[18] Cui X, Zhao Z, Zhang T, Guo W, Guo W, Zheng J, et al. A systematic review and meta-analysis of children with coronavirus disease 2019 (COVID-19). Journal of Medical Virology;**2021**:931057-931069. DOI: 10.1002/jmv.26398

[19] Centers for Disease Control and Prevention. Coronavirus disease 2019 in children – United States. 2020. MMWR. 2020; 69. Available from: https://www.cdc.gov/mmwr/volumes/69/wr/mm6914e4.htm. [Accessed: November 17, 2022]

[20] General Directorate of Epidemiology. Secretary of Health. Update of operational definition of suspected case of viral respiratory disease. 2020. Available from: https://www.gob.mx/cms/uploads/attachment/file/573732/Comunicado_Oficial_DOC_sospechoso_ERV_240820.pdf. [Accessed: December 1, 2022]

[21] World Health Organization. Interpretation of laboratory results for COVID-19 diagnosis, 6 May 2020. 2020. Available from: https://iris.paho.org/handle/10665.2/52138. [Accessed: December 1, 2022]

[22] World Health Organization. Report of the WHO-China Joint Mission on Coronavirus Disease 2019 (COVID-19). 2020. Available from: https://www.who.int/publications-detail/report-of-the-who-china-joint-mission-on-coronavirus-disease-2019-(covid-19). [Accessed: December 1, 2022]

[23] Livingston E, Bucher K. Coronavirus disease 2019 (COVID-19) in Italy. Journal of the American Medical Association. 2020;**323**(14):1335. DOI: 10.1001/jama.2020.4344

[24] Tagarro A, Epalza C, Santos M, Sanza-Santaeufemia FJ, Otheo E, Moraleda C, et al. Screening and severity of Coronavirus disease 2019 (COVID-19) in children in Madrid, Spain, JAMA Pediatrics.2020;e201346. DOI: 10.1001/jamapediatrics.2020.1346

[25] Verdoni L, Mazza A, Gervasoni A, et al. An outbreak of severe Kawasaki-like disease at the Italian epicentre of the SARS-CoV-2 epidemic: An observational cohort study. Lancet. 2020;**395**(10239):1771-1778. DOI: 10.1016/S0140-6736(20)31103-X

[26] Whittaker E, Bamford A, Kenny J, et al. Clinical characteristics of 58 children with a pediatric inflammatory multisystem síndrome temporally associated with SARS-CoV-2. JAMA. 2020;**324**:259-269. DOI: 10.1001/jama.2020.10369

[27] Antúnez-Montes OY, Escamilla MI, Figueroa-Uribe AF, Arteaga-Menchaca E, Lavariega-Saráchaga M, Salcedo-Lozada P, et al. COVID-19 and multisystem inflammatory syndrome in Latin American children. A multinational study. The Pediatric Infectious Disease Journal. 2021;**40**(1):e1-e6. DOI: 10.1097/INF.0000000000002949

[28] Toubiana J, Poirault C, Corsia A, Bajolle F, Fourgeaud J, Angoulvant F, et al. Kawasaki-like multisystemic inflammatory síndrome in children during the COVID-19 pandemic in Paris, France: Prospective observational study. BMJ. 2020;**369**:m2094. DOI: 10.1136/bmj.m2094

[29] Pouletty M, Borocco C, Ouldali N, Caseris M, Basmaci R, Lachaume N, et al. Paediatric multisystem inflammatory syndrome temporally associated with SARS-CoV-2 mimicking Kawasaki disease (Kawa-COVID-19): A multicentre cohort. Annals of the Rheumatic Diseases. 2020;**79**(8):999-1006. DOI: 10.1136/annrheumdis-2020-217960

[30] Rivas-Ruiz R, Roy-García IA, Ureña-Wong KR, Aguilar-Ituarte F, Vázquez-de Anda GF, Gutiérrez-Castrellón P, et al. Factors associated with death in children with COVID-19 in Mexico. Gaceta Médica de México. 2020;**156**:516-522. DOI: 10.24875/GMM,M21000478

[31] Moreno-Noguez M, Rivas-Ruiz R, Roy-García IA, Pacheco-Rosas DO, Moreno-Espinosa S, Flores-Pulido AA. Risk factors associated with SARS-CoV-2 pneumonia in the pediatric population. Boletín Médico del Hospital Infantil de México. 2021;**75**(4):251-258. DOI: 10.24875/BMHIM.20000263

[32] Padilla-Raygoza N, Sandoval-Salazar C, Diaz-Becerril LA, Beltran-Campos V, Diaz-Martinez DA, Navarro-Olivos G-LMJ, et al. Update of the evolution of SARS-CoV-2 infection, COVID_19, and mortality in Mexico until May 15, 2020: An ecological study. International Journal of tropical disease & Health. 2020;**41**(5):36-45. DOI: 10.9734/IJTDH/2020/v41i/530277

[33] Navarro-Olivos E, Padilla-Raygoza N, Flores-Vargas G, Gallardo-Luna MDJ, León-Verdín MG, Lara-Lona E, et al. COVID-19-associated case fatality rate in subjects under 18 years old in Mexico, up to December 31, 2020. Frontiers in Pediatrics. 2021;**9**:696425. DOI: 10.3389/fped.2021.696425

[34] Atamari-Anahui N, Cruz-Nina ND, Condori-Huaraka M, Nuñez-Paucar H, Rondon-Abuhadba EA, Ordoñez-Linares ME, et al. Caracterización de la enfermedad por coronavirus 2019 (COVID-19) en niños y adolescentes en países de América Latina y El Caribe: un estudio descriptivo. Medwave. 2020;**20**(8):e8025. DOI: 10.5867/medwave.2020.08.8025

[35] Padilla-Raygoza N, Sandoval-Salazar C, Ramirez-Gomez XS, Diaz-Becerril LA, Navarro-Olivos E, Gallardo-Luna MJ, et al. Status of disease by novel coronavirus and analysis of mortality in Mexico, until July 31, 2020. JOMAHR. 2020;**5**(1):26-35

[36] Chaudhuri PK, Ak C, Prasad KN, Malakar J, Pathak A, Siddalingesha R. An observational study on clinical and epidemiological profile of pediatric patients with Coronavirus Disease 2019 (COVID-9) presenting with co-morbidities at RIMS 2019 Ranchi. Journal of Family Medicine Primary Care. 2019;**2022**(11):1493-1496. DOI: 10.4103/jfmpc.jfmpc_1447_21

[37] Tsankov BK, Allaire JM, Irvine MA, Lopez AA, Sauve LJ, Vallance BA, et al. Severe COVID-19 infection and pediatric comorbidities: A systematic review and meta-analysis. International Journal of Infectious Diseases. 2021;**103**:246-256. DOI: 10.1016/j.ijid.2020.11.163

Chapter 5

COVID-19 Epidemiology in Türkiye

Emine Aylin Yılmaz and Öner Özdemir

Abstract

The World Health Organization declared the current pandemic, known as severe acute respiratory syndrome-coronavirus 2 (SARS-CoV-2) infection, which began in China in December 2019. SARS-CoV-2 has the third highest recorded pathogenicity, with mortality rates varying from 6 to 10.5% based on comorbidity of the individual infected with the virus. Epidemiologic studies have critical importance in the fight against any disease. This chapter discusses demographic and epidemiologic literature data including age, gender, reinfection, death, and vaccination rates reported in numerous articles during the pandemic process from Türkiye.

Keywords: COVID-19, SARS-CoV-2, epidemiology, demographics, Türkiye

1. Introduction

Epidemiology is critical in the fight against any disease. Epidemiology, which is the study of how diseases spread, and why, has played a significant role in the effort to understand, contain, and respond to COVID-19. The pandemic has altered epidemiology and expanded its scope. It is a cornerstone of public health, determining health policy and evidence-based practice by identifying disease risk factors and preventive healthcare targets.

The World Health Organization (WHO) declared a coronavirus pandemic in March 2020, following the outbreak of severe acute respiratory syndrome coronavirus 2 (SARS-CoV-2) infection in Wuhan, China, in December 2019. SARS-CoV-2 is one of the members of coronavirus pathogens, e.g., SARS-CoV-1, MERS-Co-V (Middle East respiratory syndrome) with mortality rates ranging from 6 to 10.5% depending on the infected individuals [1, 2]. As long as SARS-CoV-2 continues to spread rapidly around the world, a better understanding of the underlying level of transmission and infection severity is critical for guiding the pandemic response [3].

The value of quick diagnoses has been proven by the COVID-19 pandemic.

2. Characteristics of the SARS-CoV-2 and interaction with the host

SARS-CoV-2 is the one of the single-stranded RNA viruses in Coronavirus family, which includes nearly 40 species [2].

 IntechOpen

As a result of sequencing analysis, between SARS-CoV-2 and SARS-Co-VS proteins similarity was detected up to 80%. Based on this analysis, SARS-CoV-2 is classified in the β-coronavirus cluster [2]. The SARS-CoV-2S protein has a 15-fold higher affinity for the human angiotensin-converting enzyme 2 (ACE2) receptor [4]. ACE 2 receptor as well as transmembrane protease serine 2 (TMPRSS 2) enzyme plays a role in the induction of S protein. The S protein's scission regulates the entire mechanism.

3. Transmission

The primary mode of SARS-CoV-2 transmission is person-to-person respiratory transmission [5]. It is considered to spread mainly through intimate interaction *via* respiratory particles; a virus released in respiratory secretions in an infected person coughs, sneezes, or speaks can infect another person if inhaled or comes into direct contact with mucous membranes. Transmission can also occur *via* touching contaminated surfaces.

SARS-CoV-2 has been detected in non-respiratory specimens including stool, blood, ocular secretions, but their role in transmission is unknown.

4. Incubation period

The incubation period of an infectious disease is the time between exposure to an infectious agent and the appearance of signs and symptoms of the disease. A disease's incubation period can vary greatly from person to person. Understanding the incubation period data for a novel infectious agent is useful for estimating the transmission potential and pandemic, locating active cases, assessing the effectiveness of entry screening and contact tracing, and determining the pathogen's relative infectiousness. It is assumed to have a 14-day incubation period after being exposed to the pathogen [6].

5. Cytokine storm of SARS-CoV-2 infection

The severity of SARS-CoV-2 disease is linked to cytokine storming, which occurs when IL-2R, IL-6, IL-10, and TNF-a levels rise [7]. It is linked to the development of severe alveolar damage and lung inflammation as a distinct pathological picture of acute respiratory distress syndrome [7].

6. Incidence of SARS-CoV-2 infection in Türkiye

On March 10, 2020, the first COVID-19 case was diagnosed in Türkiye. Since the outbreak's inception, the city with the highest population density in the country, Istanbul, has reported the greatest number of cases [8]. According to last data, in Türkiye, coronavirus cases 17.042.722 and 101.492 coronavirus deaths were reported (https://www.worldometers.info/coronavirus/country/turkey/).

7. Clinical findings and symptoms

SARS-CoV-2 infection causes acute and highly fatal pneumonia with fever (83–99%), dry cough (60–82%), dyspnea, and bilateral ground-glass opacity on radiological thorax imaging [9]. The severity of the disease was determined primarily by clinical features and laboratory testing and was categorized as asymptomatic infection, mild, moderate, severe, and critical disease [10].

8. Distribution by age and gender in SARS-CoV-2 infection

COVID-19 can be seen in all age groups. In elderly persons and patients suffering from chronic diseases, COVID-19 may be more severe and mortal. The number of reported cases in pediatric population and the rate of serious illness are low. COVID-19 is commonly asymptomatic in children, and it is an important matter of attention during the pandemic. This situation contributes to the spread of infection.

The infection fatality ratio is estimated to be lowest among 5- to 9-year-old children, with an increased rate by age among individuals older than 30 years [3].

In Türkiye, children account for around 1–5% of COVID-19 cases [11]. Considering SARS-CoV-2 patients, it is noteworthy that the number of pediatric patients is considerably less than adults. The first reason that comes to mind to explain this situation is ACE activity [6]. It appears that COVID-19 causes less severe disease in children than in adults. The asymptomatic, mild, or moderate disease affects an estimated 90% of pediatric patients. Even so, 6.7% of the cases were severe. Severe disease has been reported in patients younger than one year of age, including children with an underlying disease [11, 12]. Various studies on the disease management strategies in pediatric patients are being conducted. One research examined 220 pediatric COVID-19 patients, 48.2% of whom were male, with a median age of 10 years, and 9.5% of whom had underlying diseases. The authors concluded that the course of COVID-19 seemed to be mild and management strategy primarily should consist of supportive care [13].

The death rate in men is higher than in women. As an explanation for this situation, the contribution of smoking rate, consumption of alcohol rate, and other risk factors to disease severity were considered in the etiology.

9. Protection

Based on previous experience with other respiratory virus, it is critical to use personal protective equipment (PPE) on a consistent basis to reduce nosocomial transmission [14].

10. COVID-19 prevalence in healthcare workers

According to the data of the Ministry of Health, research assistant doctors (12.3%) and nurses (11.1%) had the highest seropositivity rates, respectively. It has been suggested that the reason for this may be that health workers who actively participate in patient sampling, diagnosis, and treatment have greater rates of SARS-CoV-2 exposure [15].

11. MIS-C syndrome

Multisystem inflammatory syndrome in children (MIS-C) is a rare post-infectious hyperinflammatory disorder associated with SARS-CoV-2 [16]. MIS-C syndrome should be considered as a differential diagnosis in cases where persistent fever, fatigue, hypotension, cardiac dysfunction, and gastrointestinal symptoms are prominent [17]. Referring to research done on 101 patients in Türkiye, the median time of hospitalization was reported as 10 days. In the same study, the rate of need for intensive care was reported as 37.6% and the rate of need for mechanical ventilation was reported as 10.8% [17]. Procalcitonin, C-reactive protein, international normalized ratio, D-dimer, and creatinine levels were also found to be higher in children who needed intensive care unit stay [17]. Nearly half of the patients received anticoagulants and aspirin to prevent the potential risk of thrombosis caused on by SARS-CoV-2 infection. Intravenous immunoglobulin was applied to treat the majority of patients; the dosage was 2 g/kg in 82% of cases and 4 g/kg in 10%. Echocardiography was performed in 85 patients and abnormal findings were noted in 45 (52.9%) patients [17].

12. Anosmia

Anosmia and ageusia are particular symptoms reported in COVID-19 patients. According to the data obtained by examining a large case series across Türkiye, anosmia (43.3%) and ageusia (44.5%) were frequently observed after general symptoms [18]. There is no definitive treatment regimen specified in the guidelines against anosmia associated with COVID-19. It was observed that anosmia resolved at a rate of 91.6% [18].

13. Vitamin D status

As a result of the study conducted with 155 participants (COVID-19 patients n:75, control group n:80) in Türkiye, mean vitamin D level was greater in the control group than the COVID-19 patient group [19]. There are other study results confirming this situation [20]. Patients with low vitamin D levels experienced greater instances of respiratory distress, weakness, anosmia, headache, myalgia, and ageusia but significantly lower instances of fever and cough [19]. Comparing the low vitamin D group to the normal vitamin D group, the mean lymphocyte count was considerably lower in the low vitamin D group [19]. The number of days of hospitalization was negatively correlated with vitamin D levels [19].

14. Mental health

In order to establish COVID-19 precautions in Türkiye, a scientific committee was set up. The day following the first case was announced, on March 12, all schools and institutions were closed. Online education for students was quickly put in place. Anxiety brought on by COVID-19 has affected everyone's mental health. During the lockdown, people began to experience tension in their relationships with others as a result of increasing anxiety. As people attempt to adjust to the new circumstances, a variety of different behaviors have been reported. These behaviors include communication issues between spouses, conflict between parents and children, an increase in irritability and outbursts, depressive and anxious moods, excessive use of social media, and binge eating. Additionally, eating and sleeping habits significantly disturbed [21].

15. COVID-19 incidence in chronic disease patients in Türkiye

At least one-quarter of patients with COVID-19 have one of the chronic diseases as a comorbidity such as diabetes mellitus, hypertension, and asthma [22]. In a Turkish study, the most common comorbidities were hypertension (9.1%), diabetes (7.6%), and coronary artery disease (6.9%) [23].

16. Mortality in Türkiye

In Türkiye, which has a powerful health system, the majority of hospitals have been converted into pandemic hospitals, scheduled procedures have been postponed, and medical professionals have been reassigned to treat COVID-19. According to study, the overall mortality rate was 1.4% [23]. Re-infection caused death in 2% of the cases [23].

17. What is a reinfection and how are the rates in Türkiye?

A reinfection occurs when an individual becomes infected with COVID-19, recovers, passes a certain amount of time, and later becomes infected again. If a person tests positive again in ≥90 days after their first-positive SARS-CoV-2 RT-PCR test, they are considered to have been reinfected. The study included 58,811 patients diagnosed with COVID-19 between March 2020 and August 2021. Re-infection rate was reported in 421 patients (0, 7%) [23]. The cases had an average age of 38.0 ± 16.0 years, with 51% of them being female. About 17.6% of all re-infected cases were healthcare workers. The prevalence of chronic diseases was reported to be 31.1% [23]. While the hospitalization rate for the first infection was 15.9%, it was 9.1% for re-infection. The re-infection admission rate to the intensive care unit was higher (2.9%), than the first infection (0.5%) [23].

18. Vaccination in Türkiye

The SARS-CoV-2 pandemic, which started in 2019, has been a very difficult global pandemic process. Vaccination is among the most effective public health interventions that modern medicine has to offer [24]. Vaccination is regarded as the most important tool in controlling the pandemic [25].

In addition to vaccination, vitamin D supplementation plays an important role in immune system modulation by suppressing proinflammatory cytokines [26, 27]. There were no hospitalizations or deaths among fully vaccinated patients. Furthermore, none of the fatal cases had completed their vaccination schedule [23].

Unvaccinated individuals make about 2/3 of re-infection cases. About 5.6% of cases were fully vaccinated. In fully vaccinated patients, no hospitalization or mortality was observed. Some of them, which were fully vaccinated, were performed a chest CT and had no radiological sign was found in any of them [23].

Author details

Emine Aylin Yılmaz[1] and Öner Özdemir[2]*

1 Department of Pediatrics, Kocaali State Hospital, Sakarya, Türkiye

2 Division of Pediatric Allergy and Immunology, Sakarya University Medical Faculty, Sakarya, Türkiye

*Address all correspondence to: ozdemir_oner@hotmail.com

IntechOpen

References

[1] Kouhpayeh S, Shariati L, Boshtam M, Rahimmanesh I, Mirian M, Zeinalian M, et al. The molecular story of COVID-19; NAD+ depletion addresses all questions in this infection. Preprints. 2020:2020030346. DOI: 10.20944/preprints202003.0346.v1

[2] Lombardy Section Italian Society Infectious and Tropical Diseases. Vademecum for the treatment of people with COVID-19. Edition 2.0, 13 March 2020. Le Infezioni in Medicina. 1 Jun 2020;**28**(2):143-152. PMID: 32275256 [Ahead of print]

[3] O'Driscoll M, Ribeiro Dos Santos G, Wang L, Cummings DAT, Azman AS, Paireau J, et al. Age-specific mortality and immunity patterns of SARS-CoV-2. Nature. 2021;**590**(7844):140-145. DOI: 10.1038/s41586-020-2918-0

[4] Zhang H, Penninger JM, Li Y, Zhong N, Slutsky AS. Angiotensin-converting enzyme 2 (ACE2) as a SARS-CoV-2 receptor: Molecular mechanisms and potential therapeutic target. Intensive Care Medicine. 2020;**46**(4):586-590. DOI: 10.1007/s00134-020-05985-9

[5] Meyerowitz EA, Richterman A, Gandhi RT, Sax PE. Transmission of SARS-CoV-2: A review of viral, host, and environmental factors. Annals of Internal Medicine. Jan 2021;**174**(1):69-79. DOI: 10.7326/M20-5008

[6] Yılmaz EA, Özdemir Ö. SARS-CoV-2 Enfeksiyonunda Patofizyoloji ve İmmün Sistemin Rolünün Klinik Bulgular ve Tedaviye Yansımaları. Sakarya Tıp Dergisi. 2022;**12**(1):178-187. DOI: 10.31832/smj.733804

[7] Costela-Ruiz VJ, Illescas-Montes R, Puerta-Puerta JM, Ruiz C, Melguizo-Rodríguez L. SARS-CoV-2 infection: The role of cytokines in COVID-19 disease. Cytokine & Growth Factor Reviews. 2020;**54**:62-75. DOI: 10.1016/j.cytogfr.2020.06.001

[8] Kepenekli E, Yakut N, Ergenc Z, Aydiner Ö, Sarinoğlu RC, Karahasan A, et al. COVID-19 disease characteristics in different pediatric age groups. Journal of Infection in Developing Countries. 2022;**16**(1):16-24. DOI: 10.3855/jidc.15353

[9] Özdemir Ö. Coronavirus disease 2019 (COVID-19): Diagnosis and management (narrative review). Erciyes Medical Journal. 2020;**42**(3):242-247. DOI: 10.14744/etd.2020.99836

[10] Karbuz A, Akkoc G, Bedir Demirdag T, Yilmaz Ciftdogan D, Ozer A, Cakir D, et al. Epidemiological, clinical, and laboratory features of children with COVID-19 in Turkey. Frontiers in Pediatrics. 2021;**9**:631547. DOI: 10.3389/fped.2021.631547

[11] Tezer H, Bedir Demirdağ T. Novel coronavirus disease (Covid-19) in children. Turkish Journal of Medical Sciences. 2020;**50**(SI-1):592-603. DOI: 10.3906/SAG-2004-174

[12] Çiftçiler R, Haznedaroğlu İC, Tufan A, Öztürk MA. Covid-19 scientific publications from Turkey. Turkish Journal of Medical Sciences. 2021;**51**(3):877-889. DOI: 10.3906/sag-2010-261

[13] Cura Yayla BC, Ozsurekci Y, Aykac K, Derin P, Lacinel Gürlevik S, Ilbay SG, et al. Characteristics and management of children with COVID-19 in Turkey. Balkan Medical Journal. 2020;**37**(6):341-347. DOI: 10.4274/balkanmedj.galenos.2020.2020.7.52

[14] Nguyen LH, Drew DA, Graham MS, Joshi AD, Guo CG, Ma W, et al. Risk of COVID-19 among front-line health-care workers and the general community: A prospective cohort study. The Lancet Public Health. 2020;**5**(9):e475-e483. DOI: 10.1016/S2468-2667(20)30164-X

[15] Yılmaz EA, Özdemir Ö. Solid organ transplantations and COVID-19 disease. World Journal of Transplantation. 2021;**11**(12):503-511. DOI: 10.5500/WJT.V11.I12.503

[16] Patel JM. Multisystem inflammatory syndrome in children (MIS-C). Current Allergy and Asthma Reports. 2022;**22**(5):53-60. DOI: 10.1007/s11882-022-01031-4

[17] Törün SH, Çiftdoğan DY, Kara A. Multisystem inflammatory syndrome in children. Turkish Journal of Medical Sciences. 2021;**51**(SI-1):3273-3283. DOI: 10.3906/sag-2105-342

[18] Elvan-Tuz A, Karadag-Oncel E, Kiran S, Kanik-Yuksek S, Gulhan B, Hacimustafaoglu M, et al. Prevalence of anosmia in 10.157 pediatric COVID-19 cases: Multicenter study from Turkey. Journal of Bone and Joint Surgery. 2022;**41**(6):473-477. DOI: 10.1097/INF.0000000000003526

[19] Alpcan A, Tursun S, Kandur Y. Vitamin D levels in children with COVID-19: A report from Turkey. Epidemiology and Infection. 2021;**149**:e180. DOI: 10.1017/S0950268821001825

[20] Yılmaz K, Şen V. Is vitamin D deficiency a risk factor for COVID-19 in children? Pediatric Pulmonology. 2020;**55**(12):3595-3601. DOI: 10.1002/ppul.25106

[21] Öğütlü H. Turkey's response to COVID-19 in terms of mental health. Irish Journal of Psychological Medicine. 2020;**37**(3):222-225. Cambridge University Press. DOI: 10.1017/ipm.2020.57

[22] Guan WJ, Liang WH, Zhao Y, Liang HR, Chen ZS, Li YM, et al. Comorbidity and its impact on 1590 patients with COVID-19 in China: A nationwide analysis. European Respiratory Society. 14 May 2020;**55**(5):2000547. DOI: 10.1183/13993003.00547-2020

[23] Arslan Y, Akgul F, Sevim B, Varol ZS, Tekin S. Re-infection in COVID-19: Do we exaggerate our worries? European Journal of Clinical Investigation. 2022;**52**(6):e13767. DOI: 10.1111/eci.13767

[24] Özdemir Ö, Aylin Yılmaz E. Management of allergic diseases during pandemic. In: Allergic Disease-New Developments in Diagnosis and Therapy [Working Title]. London, UK: IntechOpen; 2023. DOI: 10.5772/intechopen.110342

[25] Zee ST, Kwok LF, Kee KM, Fung LH, Luk WP, Chan TL, et al. Impact of COVID-19 vaccination on healthcare worker infection rate and outcome during SARS-CoV-2 omicron variant outbreak in Hong Kong. Vaccine. 2022;**10**(8):1322. DOI: 10.3390/vaccines10081322

[26] Gotelli E, Paolino S, Soldano S, Cutolo M. Vitamin D immune-mediated responses and SARS-CoV-2 infection: Clinical implications in COVID-19. Immuno. 2021;**2**(1):1-12. DOI: 10.3390/immuno2010001

[27] Kaya MO, Pamukcu E, Yakar B. The role of vitamin D deficiency on COVID-19: A systematic review and meta-analysis of observational studies. Epidemiology and Health. 2021;**43**:e2021074. DOI: 10.4178/epih.e2021074

Section 4

Clinico-Pathological Factors

Chapter 6

4-Hydroxynonenal Is Linked to Sleep and Cognitive Disturbances in Children: Once upon the Time of COVID-19

Sherine Abdelmissih

Abstract

The better prognosis of COVID-19 in children conferred a higher survival rate, but a higher prevalence of post-COVID sequalae, including insomnia and defective cognition. COVID-19 triggered oxidative stress, with hyperlipidemia correlated with susceptibility to severe COVID-19. Consequently, lipids peroxidation could be a likely candidate for disease progression and sequalae. Hence, this overview explored one of the commonly studied lipid peroxides, 4-hydroxynonenal (4-HNE), in terms of gamma-amino butyric acid (GABA) and glutamate. Higher glutamate and lower glutamine, a GABA substrate, triggered severe COVID-19. Increased glutamate and inflammatory cytokines induced GABA endocytosis, reducing the anti-inflammatory and antioxidant effects of GABA. Defective glutathione antioxidant was detected in Down syndrome, the latter was associated with severe COVID-19. Increased 4-HNE, due to consumption of electronic devices and flavors containing 1-bromopropane, was increased in inflammatory neurologic disorders. A higher hippocampal 4-HNE triggered excitotoxicity and cognitive deficits. Hippocampal inflammation and loss were also evident in COVID-19. 4-HNE might play role in disturbing sleep and cognition in children during COVID-19, a hypothesis that could be verified in future research by redeeming 4-HNE in the sputum and urine of children. Currently, supplying children with optimum dietary antioxidants, while rationalizing the use of flavors is to be encouraged.

Keywords: COVID-19, insomnia, 4-Hydroxynonenal, cognition, GABA, lipid peroxidation

1. Introduction

Until early January 2023, over 660 million cases were diagnosed with coronavirus disease (COVID-19), most cases residing in Europe with much less cases in Africa, and the United States being the most affected country [1]. When first recognized in late 2019 and early 2020, COVID-19 was thought of as an 'adult and older' disease, exempting the younger population. Later, this revelation was falsified by positive infected cases found among neonates and children. Despite lower death rates at

IntechOpen

younger ages, COVID-19 survivors are mainly those in the pediatric age group. The milder disease was related to lower immune responses in children [2].

Knowing that COVID-19 has affected 6.3% of children aged 5–14 years old from December 30, 2019 till September 13, 2022 [3] would give us clues about the magnitude of post-COVID in children, even if definite evidence is still missing [4]. Reports outlining the possibility of asymptomatic disease occurring in children [5] suggest that the global prevalence of COVID in children may be much higher than the registered cases. In contrast, other studies highlighted that children were especially afflicted by hyperinflammatory multisystem syndrome [6–8]. The issue arose when some studies detected that recurrent infection is likely to occur in school children, compared to pre-school age, and that some of the affected children tested negative for viral antigen and antibodies and they did not shed the virus [9–11], which can lead us to infinite unexplored areas of research targeting whether the virus remains dormant or not, for how long and where, in the neurological system and/or elsewhere. Are there late-onset sequalae that could affect the future quality of life of young generations or even be transmitted to their offspring after decades? The anonymous fate of viral infection in children who survived but did not shed the virus should draw the attention of investigators toward the outcomes of COVID-19 on various aspects, including cognition as one crucial vector in childhood determining the ability to learn, develop new skills, and have a future fruitful life.

During the post-COVID period, survivors suffered neuropsychiatric symptoms, including anxiety and mood disturbances [12]. Such neuropsychiatric sequalae were attributed to the viral invasion of the brain [13] and neural control over the immune system [14]. In their retrospective cohort study, Taquet, Geddes, et al. [15] noticed a higher liability for insomnia during 6 months post-COVID, one plausible explanation was the impact of inflammatory cytokines over neuroendocrine sleep mediators [16].

Although a direct link between insomnia and liability for a more severe COVID-19 was not conclusive, yet inferences could be made based on previous studies showing that persons who had less than 7 hours of daily sleeping were three times more vulnerable to getting a flu attack [17]. An association between disturbed sleep or even prolonged sleep and a state of low-grade systemic inflammation was suggested [18, 19], the latter impaired the immune defenses against the respiratory pathogens [16, 20, 21], added to a higher risk of developing pneumonia [22]. The deleterious effects of disturbed sleep over immunity were also emphasized in Module 2 of The National Institute for Occupational Safety and Health (NIOSH) [23] declaring more than 50% decline in the production of antibodies following influenza vaccination in presence of sleep shifting, compared to regular sleep.

As the susceptibility to COVID-19 is higher with cardiovascular diseases, diabetes mellitus (DM), and obesity, and as dyslipidemia is common among these vulnerable groups [24–26], a causal relationship might exist between lipid metabolism and COVID-19 morbidity. Apart from the structural, non-structural, and accessory proteins identified for severe acute respiratory syndrome virus (SARS-CoV-2), lipid-based structures remain to be identified, especially when knowing their pivotal role in viral fusion, entry, and replication and that the host lipid profile is altered following COVID-19 [27, 28]. The involvement of lipids in promoting the creation of severe acute respiratory syndrome (SARS-CoV-2) progeny is becoming increasingly an interesting entity that awaits further exploration. Interestingly, insomnia has been reported to alter lipid metabolism and trigger lipid peroxidation [29]. Both insomnia and lipid peroxidation were associated with cognitive decline [30, 31]. In this context, this overview will focus on the relationship between COVID-19, insomnia, and

4-hydroxynonenal (4-HNE), as the most studied among lipid peroxides, on one side, and cognitive defects, on the other side.

2. COVID-19 in children: insomnia and cognitive defects

The American Academy of Sleep Medicine [32] has quoted from the Centers of Disease Control (CDC) that sleep disturbances among middle- and high-school students were highly prevalent. This prevalence was also noticed in survivors of COVID-19 who experienced long-term insomnia [33] with younger age being more vulnerable [34]. During COVID-19, higher liability to insomnia was also reported in students, compared to workers, and in undergraduates, compared to postgraduates [35, 36].

Novel stressors were superimposed with the emergence of COVID-19, including locking down at home, studying in an isolated environment with no social interactions, lacking friends, missing both physical activities and teamwork-based learning, having one or more of beloved family members affected, added to dealing with stressed parents [37]. Learning at home has posed a greater stressful challenge to parents whose anxiety was transferred to their children [38]. All these stressors contributed to higher anxiety in children, and subsequent sleep issues [39], including, inability to fall asleep, insufficient duration of sleep, excessive sleep duration, nightmares, and unstable sleep timings. In turn, disturbed sleep, by triggering mood swings, caused a further reduction in social interactions [40], and impaired psychological and physical well-being [41]. Interestingly, being home alone, using electronic devices during studying, playing, or chatting, were associated with poor sleep quality in children with autism spectrum disorder (ASD) [42].

Attention, as one of the cognitive domains, tended to decline with insomnia. Focused attention, detected by responding to a specific stimulus while overlooking other stimuli, was reduced with insomnia [43]. Vigilance (sustained attention) or the ability to keep alertness over time [44] was negatively affected by insomnia with reduced accuracy and prolonged time needed to perform vigilance-related tasks [45]. Similarly, shifting attention or the ability to adapt and modify the focus of attention, requiring a higher level of cognition [46], was defective in cases with insomnia [47]. However, some other studies did not prove these correlations, especially for the simplest form of attention, focused attention [48, 49].

Another cognitive domain, memory, was negatively impacted by insomnia [50, 51], whether working memory or that of the implicit (procedural) or explicit (declarative) categories. These three memory categories correspond to the inability of keeping information for a short period [46], learning new skills, and recalling a new learned material after a delay, respectively [52]. In a meta-analysis, there was a mild correlation between insomnia and working memory, yet the authors declared that results could be biased by the heterogenicity between studied groups in different studies. Other studies denied such an insomnia-memory relationship [48, 53].

Whatever is the magnitude of controversy regarding the correlation between insomnia and cognitive defects, most studies agreed about the correlation between stress and both cognition [54, 55] and sleep, especially, at a young age [56].

What links cognition to sleep at the neuronal level? In terms of memory, the role of glutamate, the main excitatory neurotransmitter in the brain, in the encoding and consolidation of memory through binding to its ionotropic receptors, N-methyl-D-aspartate (NMDA), and its metabotropic receptors (mGLuRs), respectively, has been established [57, 58]. Li et al. [59] in a meta-analysis of the African population concluded that the higher glutamate, and the lower its byproduct, glutamine, the more severe would be COVID-19 and related cognitive defects.

In astrocytes, glutamate is converted by glutamine synthetase to glutamine, the substrate of both gamma-aminobutyric acid (GABA) and glutamate [60]. GABA, the main inhibitory neurotransmitter in the mammalian brain, is also modulated, through NMDA activation when glutamate is released, then presynaptic auto-receptors $GABA_B$ stimulation, mediating GABA endocytosis [61]. In the brain, more than 50% of synapses are GABAergic [62], signifying the pleiotropic effects of GABA.

3. Gamma-aminobutyric acid linking sleep and cognition

GABA is an amino acid present in plants, bacteria, fungi, animals, and humans [63–65]. GABA in vertebrates is synthesized and metabolized (as shown in **Figure 1**) [66, 67].

GABA acts on two types of receptors, the fast ionotropic or ligand-gated ion channel, $GABA_A$, and the slow metabotropic or G protein-coupled receptor, $GABA_B$. The binding of GABA to $GABA_A$ results in chloride influx and a fast hyperpolarization of postsynaptic neurons. While $GABA_B$ receptors are present in presynaptic and postsynaptic [68]. Postsynaptic $GABA_B$ stimulation produces a slow, but long-term hyperpolarization. Presynaptic $GABA_B$ activation reduces the release of many neurotransmitters, including GABA itself, yielding either an excitatory or inhibitory brain signaling, depending on whether the suppressed neurotransmitter was

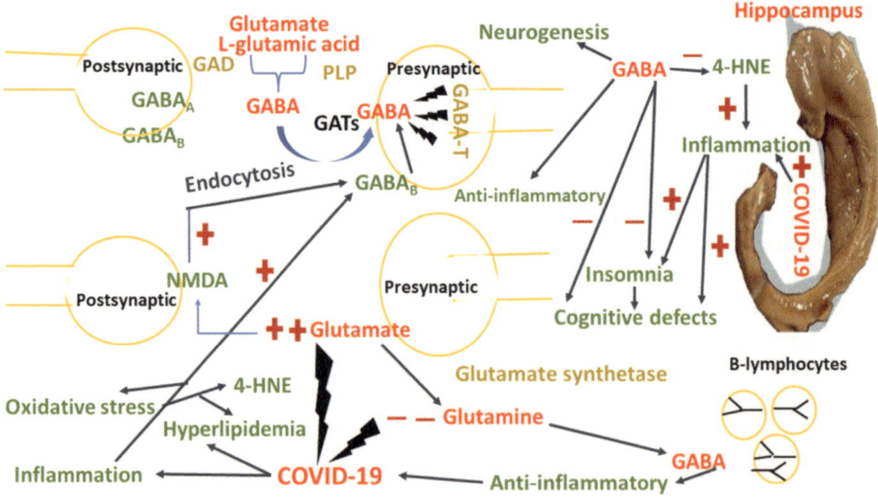

Figure 1.
GABA, glutamate, 4-HNE in COVID-19-related insomnia and cognitive defects. GABA in vertebrates is derived from L-glutamic acid or its salts, glutamate, by a decarboxylation reaction, catalyzed by GAD, and using PLP as a cofactor. After its release, GABA is uptaken by GATs 1, 2, and 3 as well as BGT-1 and metabolized by GABA-transaminases (GABA-T). Upon glutamate release, it simulates NMDA, with subsequent presynaptic $GABA_B$ activation, mediating GABA endocytosis. Increased glutamate, along with reduced glutamine, aggravates COVID severity. GABA is secreted from B-lymphocytes to exert anti-inflammatory effects. GABA promotes antioxidants, reducing lipid peroxides, including 4-HNE. COVID-19 triggers inflammation and oxidative stress. Both COVID-19 and increased hippocampal 4-HNE cause inflammation and neurodegeneration, precipitating insomnia and cognitive decline, which could be antagonized by GABA anti-inflammatory and neurogenesis effects. GABA: Gamma-aminobutyric acid; GAD: Glutamic acid decarboxylase; PLP: Pyridoxal 5'-phosphate; GATs: GABA transporters; BGT' Betaine GABA transporter; GABA-T: GABA-transaminases; Fe^{3+}: Ferric; GSH: Glutathione; NMDA: N-methyl-D-aspartate; 4-HNE: 4-Hydroxynonenal; COVID-19: Coronavirus disease.

inhibitory or excitatory. This means that if auto-receptors' presynaptic $GABA_B$ is stimulated, GABA release is dampened leading to a depolarizing postsynaptic current, or disinhibition. If a heteroreceptor $GABA_B$ was activated, glutamate release could be suppressed, which would favor an inhibitory status [69].

From functional perspective, GABA is implicated in sleep regulation and memory enhancement [70]. GABA deficiency can lead to insomnia, anxiety, and impaired stress responses [71–73]. The established role of GABA in sleep and sedation led to the wide use of benzodiazepines (BZs) as hypnotics and anxiolytics, acting by enhancing the binding of GABA to its receptors, $GABA_A$ [74, 75]. Unfortunately, BZs are associated with a high risk of tolerance and dependence [76] which mitigated their long-term use.

Despite the crucial role of GABA in the processes of sleep and cognition, it is not the only one, as inflammatory factors seem to contribute as well. In COVID-19, during the cytokine storm, excessive amounts of pro-inflammatory cytokines are produced, of which the tumor necrosis factor-alpha (TNF-α) induced the endocytosis of $GABA_A$, possibly rationalizing the associated sleep disturbances.

In the cognition domain, fast-spike GABAergic interneurons play a crucial role in the generation of electroencephalographic gamma rhythms [77], as well as hippocampal theta rhythm, corresponding to exploratory behavior [78]. Inhibitory postsynaptic potentials (IPSPs), generated by GABA, assist memory acquisition in rodents and humans [79, 80], and the progression to memory consolidation requires $GABA_B$ activation [81]. This GABA-cognitive function was experimentally verified when the passive avoidance learning of mice and rats was inhibited after the blockade of $GABA_B$ using baclofen [82, 83].

Furthermore, by promoting neurogenesis, GABA enriches long-term memory and learning processing [84]. This was emphasized in stressful conditions when mice with depressive-like symptoms exhibited defective neurogenesis and reduced microglia [85], along with reduced survival in neural stem progenitor cell culture [86]. In ASD, decreased glutamic acid decarboxylase (GAD), $GABA_{A,}$ and $GABA_B$ were observed in postmortem specimens [87], with $GABA_A$ reduction possibly underlying the co-existing delayed linguistic abilities [88], along with behavioral deficits; the latter being also demonstrated in transgenic animal models [89].

Although multiple sclerosis (MS) is mainly a disease of young adults, it is the most common neurologic disorder due to immunologic dysfunction in children and adolescents [90]. In MS, where 65% of patients have disturbed memory and attention, low plasma GABA was detected [91]. Recent reports revealed aggravated or de novo symptoms of MS associated with COVID-19 [92]. Hence, GABA might be a likely candidate for COVID-related cognitive derangement.

4. Inflammation, oxidative stress, and GABA: key targets in COVID

A growing body of evidence supports the secretion of GABA and its precursors, glutamine, and glutamate, from murine and human B-lymphocytes, [93]. While $GABA_A$ reduces T-cell response to antigens [94] and dampens inflammation, it endorses regulatory T-cells [95]. In turn, T-cells enhance the expression of GABA receptor subunits [96]. Additionally, GABA transporter-1 (GAT-1), found only on antigen-primed T-cells, arrested the proliferation of CD4+ and CD8+ T-cells [97]. Such GABA immunomodulatory effect could prevent the tissue damage elicited by inflammatory responses in cases of autoimmune diseases, as inferred from rodent models of

DM and MS [98–100]. In patients with DM, the secretion of TNF-α and interleukin (IL)-6 (IL-6) from T-cells was successfully inhibited using GABA [101, 102].

Such systemic anti-inflammatory potentiality of GABA was detected also in macrophages and dendritic cells of rodents and humans, expressing the respective fast $GABA_A$ and slow $GABA_B$ receptors [103]. GATs dampen the functions and release of pro-inflammatory cytokines as demonstrated in a mouse model of autoimmune encephalomyelitis (EAE) [97]. Thus, it was not surprising to find that the most common subtype of $GABA_A$ in the brain, (α1β2γ2), was also expressed in immune cells [104]. Conversely, immuno-stimulation and cytokines release promoted the neuronal sequestration of extracellular GABA [67]. In the brain, neuroinflammation, vascular insufficiency, and the pro-inflammatory cytokines, such as TNF-α, interferon-gamma (IFN-γ), IL-6 and IL-1β enhanced GAT expression, favoring GABA degradation [105–108].

In the context of lung diseases, GABA, along with enhanced $GABA_A$ and $GABA_B$ activities could limit acute lung injury in rodent models and ameliorate clinical outcomes in humans on ventilation [109, 110]. As an inhibitor of platelet aggregation, GABA, by inhibiting the formation of the thromboxane A2 [111], might have an additional clinical privilege in patients whose pulmonary thrombosis is attributed to the severe COVID-19 [112, 113]. These assumed benefits of early treatment with GABA in COVID-19 were verified in mice infected with mouse hepatitis virus (MHV-1) [114], another coronavirus whose symptoms mimic those of COVID-19 [115].

The COVID-associated anxiety and stress could have resulted in lowered immunity [116], which could be reversed using GABA as was emphasized in human volunteers when oral GABA administration resulted in electroencephalographic evidence of relaxed alertness and anti-stress effects (higher alpha-to-lower beta) [117], while increasing salivary IgA [118], as a non-invasive index of enhanced upper respiratory immunity against bacteria and viruses [119].

Interestingly, extracellular glutamine, the GABA precursor, was implicated in viral replication of both DNA and RNA viruses to which SARS-CoV-2 belongs, by incorporation into the Kreb's cycle after conversion by glutaminase (GLS) to alpha-ketoglutarate (α-KG), so that the lack of glutamine hampered rhinoviruses replication [120]. Presumably, if GABA synthesis is inhibited, glutamine would be redirected to promote viral replication and, in case of viral infection, defective GABA synthesis would be anticipated secondary to the incorporation of glutamine in the viral replication cycle.

Knowing that COVID-19 can precipitate oxidative stress [121, 122] while GABAergic neurons are especially susceptible to the neuro-damaging effects of the reactive oxygen species (ROS), generated during oxidative stress [123], makes both GABA and oxidative stress likely candidates for aggravating the sequalae of COVID-19.

Hypercholesterolemia might perpetuate viral infections as was the case in mice infected with lymphocyte choriomeningitis virus (LCMV) [124]. Some viral infections and related treatments can induce long-term changes in lipid metabolism as well. After 12 years of SARS-CoV, survivors had higher cell membrane phospholipids, namely, phosphatidylinositol and lysophosphatidylinositol, attributed to corticosteroid administration during the infection [125]. In the post-infection period of SARS-CoV, lysocardiolipin acetyltransferase (LCLAT), phosphoinositide phosphatase (PIP), and diacylglycerol (DG) kinase, enzymes involved in lipid metabolism, were upregulated [126].

Coronaviruses consume the intracellular membranes of host cells to build their own replication nests called "double-membrane vesicles (DMVs)," where it preserves its own viral proteins and robbed host factors, to ensure a suitable lipid bedding for a successful viral replication [127].

Of interest to our discussion is the increased total cholesterol (TC) in patients with COVID-19, favoring viral invasion, with a positive correlation to the severity of symptoms [93]. The lipid changes might be attributed to hypoxia and were also shared with patients having a chronic obstructive pulmonary disease (COPD) [128]. On the other hand, normal lipid metabolism seems preemptive in the context of pulmonary and neuronal disorders as sphingolipids were implicated in protection from a lung injury, added to their anti-inflammatory, anti-coagulant, along with their neuroprotective effects [129, 130]. Hyperlipidemia and oxidative stress during COVID make lipids peroxidation likely candidates for post-COVID syndrome.

5. Lipid peroxidation

Oxidative stress is conceived as an imbalance between oxidants and antioxidants, in favor of oxidation. In physiology, such oxidative stress is minimal and well-equilibrated in a process known as "the redox potential." It is noteworthy to mention that an imbalance in the antioxidant direction is deleterious and causes "reductive stress" [131].

Conversely, when the antioxidant mechanisms are overwhelmed, oxidative stress occurs. The consecutive reversible oxidative stress and irreversible oxidative damage are to be blamed for many pathologic conditions [132, 133]. With defective antioxidant mechanisms such as in the case of vitamin E (alpha-tocopherol) or vitamin C deficiency, excess reactive oxygen and nitrogen species are produced. The issue is that a propagation chain reaction perpetuates lipid peroxidation [131] as shown in (**Figure 2**). The interruption of chain reaction occurs when two free radicals are conjugated or when antioxidants break the chain.

Lipid peroxidation was formerly known for oils and fats in our diet. It involves oxidative damage to cellular structures, including cell membranes in plants and animals, causing cellular death. This destructive process includes the generation of lipid radicals, the uptake of oxygen, the re-organization of double bonds in unsaturated lipids, and the production of breakdown products such as alcohols, ketones, alkanes, aldehydes, and ethers. Lipid peroxidation results in an easily breakable cell membrane with plenty of polyunsaturated fatty acids (PUFAs) and transition metals. Lipid peroxidation reduces membrane fluidity and makes it more permissible and easily invaded. Apart from the loss of cell membrane integrity, protein synthesis is disrupted, as well as macrophage function, along with derangement of chemotactic signals and altered enzyme activity [134]. All membranes of cellular structures are damaged, including those of mitochondria, microsomes, peroxisomes, and cell membranes [135]. Lipid peroxidation toxicity affects the liver, kidneys, and to our interest, neurological structures, where it takes part in neurodegenerative, inflammatory, and infectious diseases [136].

Considering the brain as a susceptible organ to oxidative stress, the intracellular antioxidant, free glutathione (GSH) plays a crucial role by eliminating peroxides [137] in a reaction catalyzed by glutathione peroxidase (GSH-Px), oxidizing GSH to GSH disulfide (GSSG) [138]. Thus, the GSH/GSSG can be used as a determinant of the redox status of cells [139]. Defective GSH was previously correlated to Down syndrome in children [140]. Recently, Down syndrome was correlated to severe COVID-19 [141].

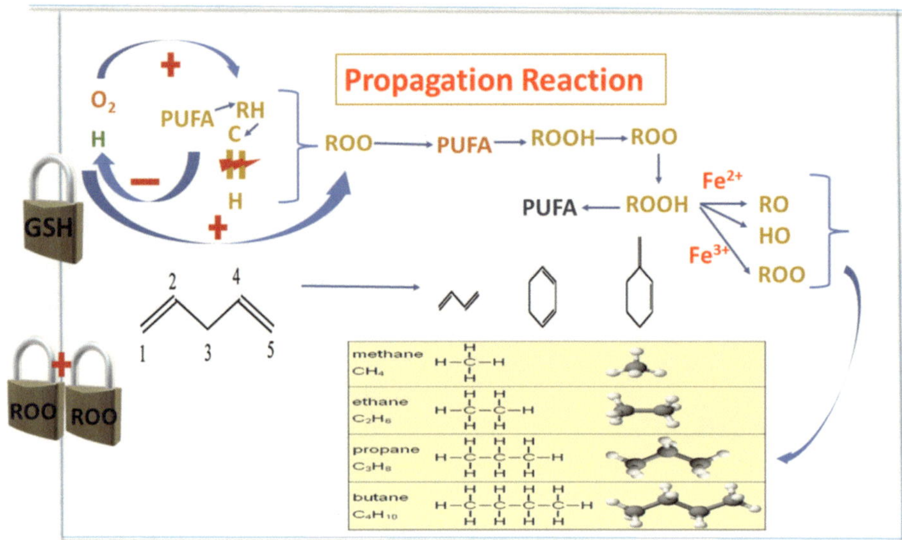

Figure 2.
Propagation reaction of lipid peroxidation. Lipid peroxidation is initiated with hydrogen subtraction and oxygen addition. Hydrogen subtraction is promoted in PUFAs by the presence of a double bond of the RH group, leaving the carbon with an unpaired electron. When combined with oxygen, ROO is produced, generating ROOH, capable of repeating the hydrogen subtraction from another PUFA, perpetuating the chain reaction. When lipid peroxides interact with Fe^{+2}, RO radicals are produced, when the interaction involves Fe^{+3}, ROO radicals are generated. These reactions will end up with cytotoxic aldehydes and hydrocarbon gases as ethane. The interruption of chain reaction occurs when two free radicals are conjugated or when antioxidants, such as GSH, break the chain. PUFA: Polyunsaturated fatty acids; RH: methylene; ROO: Peroxyl; ROOH: Hydroperoxide; Fe^{2+}: Ferrous; RO: Alcoxyl; Fe^{3+}: Ferric; GSH: Glutathione.

Most of brain GSH is derived from the reducing action of GSH reductase (GR) over GSSG to get back GSH. Another less amount of GSH can be synthesized *de novo* from glutamate, cysteine, and glycine [142].

In contrast to the antioxidant GSH, one of the lipid peroxides, 4-hydroxynonenal (4-HNE), an α, β-unsaturated aldehyde, is a potent neurotoxin, derived from the oxidation of ω-6 PUFA of cell membranes [143], such as arachidonic acid, linoleic and linolenic acid.

6. 4-Hydroxynonenal

4-Hydroxynonenal (4-HNE) is described as a short-chain reactive carbonyl compound [144], having amphiphilic properties yet with lipophilic tendency [143]. Its high electrophilicity makes it reactive to the amino acid residues, namely, cysteine (Cys), histidine (His), and lysine (Lys), in a decrescendo order. 4-HNE can adduct to the cysteine residue of the "flippase" enzyme (amino phospholipid-translocase), an enzyme that maintains lipid bilayer asymmetry by an ATP-dependent process [145]. Forming Michael adducts with nucleophilic sites, 4-HNE can interact with cellular DNA, lipids, and proteins [146]. The destiny of 4-HNE protein adducts is either proteolysis or covalent cross-linking. Additionally, 4-HNE can inactivate GR, reducing the antioxidant ability of GSH [147]. In turn, physiological concentrations of GSH can revert 4-HNE protein adducts to their unadducted condition [148].

The metabolism of 4-HNE occurs by oxidative and reductive processes, employing enzymatic and non-enzymatic pathways [144], in addition to conjugation to GSH catalyzed by the glutathione-S transferases (GST), which contributes to a major part in the detoxification process [149]. Although all these detoxifying processes are present in the mitochondria [150], yet it seems that the mitochondria play little role in 4-HNE degradation in intact tissue.

In the lungs, GST is more active than the liver, then comes the brain in the third place, however, the respiratory capacity to metabolize 4-HNE is limited by slow oxidative-reductive pathways, unlike the liver [151, 152]. 4-HNE can be detected in human breath and sputum [153] and its metabolites can be recovered in urine [154]. A slow metabolism of 4-HNE was previously reported when dealing with rat hearts and kidneys, along with other tissues [155].

To our knowledge, HNE concentration at or below 1 μM might be physiological, with in vitro toxicity at 10 μM–1 mM [156]. The physiological roles of HNE include, but are not limited to [see **Table 1**] [157–164]. Dianzani [156] mentioned that, in pathologic conditions, the high concentrations of 4-HNE suppress mitochondrial oxidation, lysosomal enzyme activity, adenyl cyclase, sodium pump, protein synthesis, and cell proliferation. Also, while physiological 4-HNE concentrations can affect proteins, favoring proteolysis of the deformed proteins [165], only extra-physiologic concentrations of 4-HNE can increase membrane fluidity [166].

In inflammatory disorders such as osteoarthritis, 20 μM HNE suppressed the high nuclear factor-kappa beta (NF-κB) induced by TNF-α overexpression in human

Targets of HNE	Role
Neutrophils chemotactic factor [157]	Increased inflammatory response to invading pathogens
AC [158]	Catalyze the breakdown of ATP to yield cAMP
PLC [159]	Hydrolysis of inositol phospholipids in cell membranes, yielding the intracellular second messengers: IP_3 and DAG
Caspases [160]	Protease enzymes that mediate programmed cell death, leading, for example, to tumor suppression and axonal degeneration
Hsp 70 [161]	Increased antigens delivery to APCs Suppression of inflammation
Aldose reductase [162]	Cytosolic NADPH-dependent oxidoreductase that catalyzes the reduction of monosaccharides, for example, the reduction of glucose to sorbitol, the first step in glucose metabolism
Hem oxygenases [163]	The degradation of heme to CO, biliverdin and heme iron, mediating anti-inflammatory, anti-apoptotic, and potential anti-viral functions
γ-GCS [164]	Catalyzes the production of γ-glutamylcysteine from both glutamate and cysteine, and other glutamylpeptides and can be used as predictor of defective GSH redox

AC: Adenyl cyclase; ATP: Adenosine triphosphate; cAMP: Cyclic adenosine monophosphate; PLC: Phospholipase C; IP_3: Inositol 1,4, 5-triphosphate; DAG: diacyl glycerol; Hsp 70: Heat shock proteins 70; APCs: Antigen-presenting cells; NADPH: Nicotinamide adenine dinucleotide phosphate hydrogen; CO: Carbon monoxide; γ-GCS: γ-glutamyl cys synthetase; GSH: Glutathione.
At physiologic concentration, HNE seems to exert immunostimulatory activity by enhancing neutrophils' chemotactic factor, increasing the production of multiple intracellular second messengers, such as cAMP, IP_3, DAG, mediate tumor suppression, and might promote axonal degeneration and aging, along with immune-stimulatory, anti-inflammatory, anti-apoptotic, and possibly anti-viral functions. HNE catalyzes glucose metabolism and interestingly, can increase antioxidant activity.

Table 1.
Physiological targets stimulated by hydroxynonenal (HNE).

osteoblasts [167]. While most studies focused on the link between 4-HNE and hepatic insult, few of them found that 4-HNE was also implicated in multiple respiratory and neurological disorders, such as bronchial asthma, COPD [168], Alzheimer's disease (AD), and Parkinson's disease (PD) [169]. The ability of 4-HNE to diffuse from one organ to another [170] might indicate the accumulation of HNE in the lungs, for instance, can affect the brain, and vice versa. Fortunately, GSH was able to suppress 4-HNE protein adducts in the liver, lungs, and brain [152].

In COPD, HNE adducts were increased in bronchial, bronchiolar, alveolar, and endothelial cells as well as macrophages and neutrophils. In alveolar epithelium, HNE adducts were inversely correlated to forced expiratory volume in 1 sec and positively linked to the pro-fibrotic cytokine, transforming growth factor-beta (TGF-β) [171]. In rat alveolar epithelial cells, HNE induced glutamylcysteinyl glycine (GCS), the rate-limiting enzyme in GSH synthesis [172], and enhanced the expression of antioxidants by recruiting nuclear factor erythroid 2-related factor-2 (Nrf2) [173, 174].

In vitro exposure to mild stress assisted the accelerated GSH-mediated removal of HNE and enhanced resistance to oxidative stress [175], which might not apply to chronic stress when antioxidants are consumed.

Measuring HNE in umbilical cord plasma, it was increased in full-term newborns exposed to acidosis and in full—as well as pre-term neonates experiencing asphyxia when compared to healthy controls [176]. A suggested role in autoimmunity was reported in children with systemic lupus erythematosus (SLE) when plasma HNE was increased, especially during the active disease stage [177].

The brain is a vulnerable organ that can be affected by oxidative stress owing to its relatively lower antioxidant capacity against a higher oxygen consumption rate, added to the abundance of PUFAs in neuronal cell membranes [178]. Upon 12-day exposure of rats to oral 1- bromopropane (1-BP), a cleaning agent for electronic and optical instruments and an intermediate in the synthesis of pharmaceuticals and flavors, the animals demonstrated behavioral evidence of impaired cognition with underlying oxidative stress as shown by the reduced level of GSH versus increased GSSG, owing to the inhibitory effect of 1-BP over GR, with subsequently increased 4-hydroxynonenal (4-HNE) and malondialdehyde (MDA) [179]. The increased 4-HNE was also replicated in patients with AD showing mild cognitive dysfunction [180]. It is to be noted that while human exposure to 1-BP is by inhalation, yet, in experimental animals, the inhalation route might not yield similar neurological effects as the oral route.

4-HNE can form adducts with glutamate transporter, excitatory amino acid transporter 2 (EAAT2) [181], dopamine transporter, sodium pump [182], dopamine 1 (D1)-like transporter [183], and immunoglobulins [184]. In cultured rat cerebrocortical neurons, HNE uncoupled cholinergic and glutamatergic receptors from the GTP-binding proteins [185]. In patients with ischemia–reperfusion and stroke, plasma HNE was elevated [186]. Immunohistochemical assay of the brain lesions in patients with the progressive demyelinating disease, multiple sclerosis, and the dominant autosomal disorder, Huntington's disease (HD), detected increased HNE [187, 188], along with elevation of the inflammatory marker C-reactive protein in serum of patients with advanced HD. In rat hippocampal cell culture, 10 μM HNE hampered sodium pump activity, resulting in increased intracellular free Ca^{2+} and predisposition to excitotoxicity [189]. The hippocampus is well known for its relevance to both cognition [190, 191] and insomnia-related cognitive issues at all ages, including children [192, 193], and inflammation and loss were recently reported in COVID-19 [194].

7. Hydroxynonenal- and GABA-targeted therapies

Based on the presumptive involvement of HNE in COVID-related insomnia and subsequent cognitive dysfunction, HNE-targeted therapy might offer an exit doorway that might rescue the young generation. For instance, carnosine, a dipeptide (β-alanyl-L-histidine) abundant in mammalian skeletal muscle, can inhibit the cross-linking of HNE protein adducts [195], and its analogs showed a similar neuroprotective effect as emphasized in rats [196].

Nutritional support seems crucial to sustaining the growth and development of childhood processes, including those related to their emotional, cognitive, and behavioral aspects. Above all, supplying dietary antioxidants, including vitamin E, vitamin C, and glutathione, could be helpful. The consumption of wheat germ oil, sunflower oil and seeds, hazelnuts, and peanut butter, as sources of vitamin E, and red and green pepper, orange, kiwi, and broccoli, providing vitamin C, with recommended daily dietary allowances at 4–13 years old of 7–11 and 25–45 mg, respectively [197].

Despite the controversies regarding the extent of systemic GABA to cross the BBB [198–200] as quoted by Tian et al. [114], supplying dietary GABA could add some benefit as an adjuvant to COVID treatment, especially since GABA has antioxidant properties [201, 202], GABA can be obtained from tomatoes, rice, soybean, and fermented food [70]. It is worthwhile that this policy can be adopted in the context of cognitive affection in children whose anxiety and insomnia could be the major contributing factors to the post-COVID syndrome.

8. Conclusion

Lipid peroxidation, along with inflammatory crisis, plays a crucial role, not only in the prognosis of COVID-19 but also in neurological sequalae, namely, sleep and cognitive issues, by affecting both GABA and glutamate neurotransmission.

4-HNE might have some role in both COVID-19 and its neurological sequalae, triggering hippocampal inflammation and neurodegeneration, by disturbing glutamate/ GABA neurotransmission.

Perhaps a nutritional supply of antioxidants and abstaining from the consumption of flavors could support our children to maintain optimal sleep and develop cognitive skills. The rationale use of electronic devices is also recommended. A more vigorous investigation is still needed to verify the hypothesis of 4-HNE involvement and to explore the feasibility of GABA—and HNE-targeted therapy in children who survived COVID-19 with residual issues regarding sleep and cognition.

Conflict of interest

The author declares no conflict of interest.

Notes

- COVID-19 triggers insomnia and cognitive defects.

- Higher glutamate, with subsequent low GABA, was associated with severe COVID-19.
- Electronic Devices and flavors could lead to increased 4-HNE.
- Increased 4-HNE caused hippocampal inflammation, an area implicated in sleep and cognition.
- Supplying pediatric nutrition with antioxidants and abstaining from flavors consumption and overuse of electronic devices might prove preemptive in COVID-19, and related sleep and cognitive issues.

Author details

Sherine Abdelmissih
Faculty of Medicine, Kasr Al-Ainy, Cairo University, Cairo, Egypt

*Address all correspondence to: drshery_wa@yahoo.com; drshery_wa@kasralainy.edu.eg

References

[1] The World Health Organization (WHO). WHO coronavirus (COVID-19) dashboard. WHO Coronavirus (COVID-19) Dashboard | WHO Coronavirus (COVID-19) Dashboard with Vaccination Data. 2023 [Accessed: 10 January 2023]

[2] Dong Y, Mo X, Hu Y, Qi X, Jiang F, Jiang Z, et al. Epidemiology of COVID-19 among children in China. Pediatrics. 2020;**145**(6):e20200702. DOI: 10.1542/peds.2020-0702

[3] Hoang A, Chorath K, Moreira M, Evans M, Burmeister-Morton F, Burmeister F, et al. COVID-19 in 7780 pediatric patients: A systematic review. EClinicalMedicine. 2020;**24**:100433. DOI: 10.1016/j.eclinm.2020.100433

[4] Buonsenso D, Munblit D, De Rose C, Sinatti D, Ricchiuto A, Carfi A, et al. Preliminary evidence on long COVID in children. Acta Paediatrica. 2021;**110**(7):2208-2211. DOI: 10.1111/apa.15870

[5] Buitrago-Garcia D, Egli-Gany D, Counotte MJ, Hossmann S, Imeri H, Ipekci A, et al. Occurrence and transmission potential of asymptomatic and presymptomatic SARS-CoV-2 infections: A living systematic review and meta-analysis. PLoS Medicine. 2020;**17**(9):e1003346. DOI: 10.1371/journal.pmed.1003346

[6] Jiang L, Tang K, Levin M, Irfan O, Morris SK, Wilson K, et al. COVID-19 and multisystem inflammatory syndrome in children and adolescents. The Lancet Infectious Diseases. 2020;**20**(11):e276-e288. DOI: 10.1016/S1473-3099(20)30651-4

[7] Dufort EM, Koumans EH, Chow EJ, Rosenthal EM, Muse A, Rowlands J, et al. Multisystem inflammatory syndrome in children in New York State. The New England Journal of Medicine. 2020;**383**(4):347-358. DOI: 10.1056/NEJMoa2021756

[8] Riphagen S, Gomez X, Gonzalez-Martinez C, Wilkinson N, Theocharis P. Hyperinflammatory shock in children during COVID-19 pandemic. Lancet. 2020;**395**(10237):1607-1608. DOI: 10.1016/S0140-6736(20)31094-1

[9] Somekh E, Gleyzer A, Heller E, Lopian M, Kashani-Ligumski L, Czeiger S, et al. The role of children in the dynamics of intra family coronavirus 2019 spread in densely populated area. The Pediatric Infectious Disease Journal. 2020;**39**(8):e202-e204. DOI: 10.1097/INF.0000000000002783

[10] Yung CF, Kam KQ, Chong CY, Nadua KD, Li J, Tan NWH, et al. Household transmission of severe acute respiratory syndrome coronavirus 2 from adults to children. The Journal of Pediatrics. 2020;**225**:249-251. DOI: 10.1016/j.jpeds.2020.07.009

[11] Tosif S, Neeland MR, Sutton P, Licciardi PV, Sarkar S, Selva KJ, et al. Immune responses to SARS-CoV-2 in three children of parents with symptomatic COVID-19. Nature Communications. 2020;**11**(1):5703. DOI: 10.1038/s41467-020-19545-8

[12] Taquet M, Luciano S, Geddes JR, Harrison PJ. Bidirectional associations between COVID-19 and psychiatric disorder: Retrospective cohort studies of 62 354 COVID-19 cases in the USA. Lancet Psychiatry. 2021;**8**(2):130-140. DOI: 10.1016/S2215-0366(20)30462-4

[13] Meinhardt J, Radke J, Dittmayer C, Franz J, Thomas C, Mothes R, et al.

Olfactory transmucosal SARS-CoV-2 invasion as a port of central nervous system entry in individuals with COVID-19. Nature Neuroscience. 2020;**24**(2):168-175. DOI: 10.1038/s41593-020-00758-5

[14] Kreye J, Reincke SM, Kornau HC, Sanchez-Sendin E, Corman VM, Liu H, et al. A therapeutic non-self-reactive SARS-CoV-2 antibody protects from lung pathology in a COVID-19 Hamster model. Cell. 2020;**183**(4):1058-1069. DOI: 10.1016/j.cell.2020.09.049

[15] Taquet M, Geddes JR, Husain M, Luciano S, Harrison PJ. 6-month neurological and psychiatric outcomes in 236 379 survivors of COVID-19: A retrospective cohort study using electronic health records. Lancet Psychiatry. 2021;**8**(5):416-427. DOI: 10.1016/S2215-0366(21)00084-5

[16] Ibarra-Coronado EG, Velazquez-Moctezuma J, Diaz D, Becerril-Villanueva LE, Pavon L, et al. Sleep deprivation induces changes in immunity in Trichinella spiralis-infected rats. International Journal of Biological Sciences. 2015;**11**(8):901-912. DOI: 10.7150/ijbs.11907

[17] Cohen S, Doyle WJ, Alper CM, Janicki-Deverts D, Turner RB. Sleep habits and susceptibility to the common cold. Archives of Internal Medicine. 2009;**169**(1):62-67. DOI: 10.1001/archinternmed.2008.505

[18] Lasselin J, Rehman JU, Akerstedt T, Lekander M, Axelsson J. Effect of long-term sleep restriction and subsequent recovery sleep on the diurnal rhythms of white blood cell subpopulations. Brain, Behavior, and Immunity. 2015;**47**:93-99. DOI: 10.1016/j.bbi.2014.10.004

[19] Irwin MR, Olmstead R, Carroll JE. Sleep disturbance, sleep duration, and inflammation: A systematic review and Meta-analysis of cohort studies and experimental sleep deprivation. Biological Psychiatry. 2016;**80**(1):40-52. DOI: 10.1016/j.biopsych.2015.05.014

[20] Spiegel K, Leproult R, Van Cauter E. Impact of sleep debt on physiological rhythms. Revue Neurologique (Paris). 2003;**159**(11 Suppl):6S11-6S20. ISSN (Linking): 0035-3787

[21] Ferrie JE, Kivimaki M, Akbaraly TN, Singh-Manoux A, Miller MA, Gimeno D, et al. Associations between change in sleep duration and inflammation: Findings on C-reactive protein and interleukin 6 in the Whitehall II study. American Journal of Epidemiology. 2013;**178**(6):956-961. DOI: 10.1093/aje/kwt072

[22] Patel SR, Malhotra A, Gao X, Hu FB, Neuman MI, Fawzi WW. A prospective study of sleep duration and pneumonia risk in women. Sleep. 2012;**35**(1):97-101. DOI: 10.5665/sleep.1594

[23] The National Institute of Occupational Safety and Health (NIOSH). Centers for Disease Control AND Prevention (CDC). NIOSH Training for Nurses on Shift Work and Long Work Hours. Part 1. The Risks and Why These Occur. Module 2. How shift work and long work hours increase health and safety risks. Module 2. Sleep and the Immune System | NIOSH | CDC [Accessed: 10 January 2023]

[24] Klop B, Elte JW, Cabezas MC. Dyslipidemia in obesity: Mechanisms and potential targets. Nutrients. 2013;**5**:1218-1240. DOI: 10.3390/nu5041218

[25] Krist AH, Davidson KW, Mangione CM, Barry MJ, Cabana M, Caughey AB, et al. Behavioral counseling interventions to promote a healthy diet and physical activity for cardiovascular disease prevention in adults with

cardiovascular risk factors: US preventive services task force recommendation statement. JAMA. 2020;**324**:2069-2075. DOI: 10.1001/jama.2020.21749

[26] Savelieff MG, Callaghan BC, Feldman EL. The emerging role of dyslipidemia in diabetic microvascular complications. Current Opinion in Endocrinology Diabetes Obesity. 2020;**27**:115-123. DOI: 10.1097/MED.0000000000000533

[27] Hu X, Chen D, Wu L, He G, Ye W. Declined serum high density lipoprotein cholesterol is associated with the severity of COVID-19 infection. Clinical Chimica Acta. 2020;**510**:105-110. DOI: 10.1016/j.cca.2020.07.015

[28] Peng Y, Wan L, Fan C, Zhang P, Wang X, Sun J, et al. Cholesterol metabolism-impacts on SARS-CoV-2 infection prognosis. medRxiv. Preprint posted online August 13, 2020. DOI: 10.1101/2020.04.16.20068528

[29] Semenova NV, Madaeva IM, Kolesnikov SI, Solodova EI, Kolesnikova LI. Insomnia in peri- and postmenopausal women: Plasma lipids, lipid peroxidation and some antioxidant system parameters. Neuropsychiatry (London). 2018;**8**(4):1452-1460. DOI: 10.4172/Neuropsychiatry.1000477

[30] Reed TT. Lipid peroxidation and neurodegenerative disease. Free Radical Biology & Medicine. 2011;**51**(7):1302-1319. DOI: 10.1016/j.freeradbiomed.2011.06.027

[31] Wardle-Pinkston S, Slavish DC, Taylor DJ. Insomnia and cognitive performance: A systematic review and meta-analysis. Sleep Medicine Reviews. 2019;**48**:101205. DOI: 10.1016/j.smrv.2019.07.008

[32] The American Academy of Sleep Medicine. CDC reports that insufficient sleep is common on school nights (aasm.org). 2018 [Accessed: 13 January 2023]

[33] Choudhry AA, Shahzeen F, Choudhry SA, Batool N, Murtaza F, Dilip A, et al. Impact of COVID-19 infection on quality of sleep. Cureus. 2021;**13**(9):e18182. DOI: 10.7759/cureus.18182

[34] Mandelkorn U, Genzer S, Choshen-Hillel S, Reiter J, Meira E, Cruz M, et al. Escalation of sleep disturbances amid the COVID-19 pandemic: A cross-sectional international study. Journal of Clinical Sleep Medicine. 2021;**17**(1):45-53. DOI: 10.5664/jcsm.8800

[35] Marelli S, Castelnuovo A, Somma A, Castronovo V, Mombelli S, Bottoni D, et al. Impact of COVID-19 lockdown on sleep quality in university students and administration staff. Journal of Neurology. 2021;**268**(1):8-15. DOI: 10.1007/s00415-020-10056-6

[36] Kokou-Kpolou CK, Megalakaki O, Laimou D, Kousouri M. Insomnia during COVID-19 pandemic and lockdown: Prevalence, severity, and associated risk factors in French population. Psychiatry Research. 2020;**290**:113128. DOI: 10.1016/j.psychres.2020.113128

[37] Prime H, Andrews K, McTavish J, Harris M, Janus M, Bennett T, et al. The application of positive parenting interventions to academic school readiness: A scoping review. Child: Care, Health and Development. 2021;**47**(1):1-14. DOI: 10.1111/cch.12810

[38] Douglas KD, Smith KK, Stewart MW, Walker J, Mena L, Zhang L. Exploring Parents' intentions to monitor and mediate adolescent social media use and implications for school nurses. The Journal of School Nursing. 2020;**2020**:105. DOI: 10.1177/1059840520983286

[39] Altena E, Baglioni C, Espie CA, Ellis J, Gavriloff D, Holzinger B, et al. Dealing with sleep problems during home confinement due to the COVID-19 outbreak: Practical recommendations from a task force of the European CBT-I academy. Journal of Sleep Research. 2020;**29**(4):e13052. DOI: 10.1111/jsr.13052

[40] Wakefield JRH, Bowe M, Kellezi B, Butcher A, Groeger JA, Longitudinal associations between family identification. Loneliness, depression, and sleep quality. British Journal of Health Psychology. 2020;**25**(1):1-16. DOI: 10.1111/bjhp.12391

[41] Grossman ES, Hoffman YSG, Palgi Y, Shrira A. COVID-19 related loneliness and sleep problems in older adults: Worries and resilience as potential moderators. Personality and Individual Differences. 2021;**168**:110371. DOI: 10.1016/j.paid.2020.110371

[42] Brooks JD, Bronskill SE, Fu L, Saxena FE, Arneja J, Pinzaru VB, et al. Identifying children and youth with autism Spectrum disorder in electronic medical records: Examining health system utilization and comorbidities. Autism Research. 2021;**14**(2):400-410. DOI: 10.1002/aur.2419

[43] Vignola A, Lamoureux C, Bastien CH, Morin CM. Effects of chronic insomnia and use of benzodiazepines on daytime performance in older adults. The Journals of Gerontology. Series B, Psychological Sciences and Social Sciences. 2000;**55**(1):P54-P62. DOI: 10.1093/geronb/55.1.p54

[44] Mirsky AF, Anthony BJ, Duncan CC, Ahearn MB, Kellam SG. Analysis of the elements of attention: A neuropsychological approach. Neuropsychology Review. 1991;**2**(2):109-145. DOI: 10.1007/BF01109051

[45] Altena E, Van Der Werf YD, Strijers RL, Van Someren EJ. Sleep loss affects vigilance: Effects of chronic insomnia and sleep therapy. Journal of Sleep Research. 2008;**17**(3):335-343. DOI: 10.1111/j.1365-2869.2008.00671.x

[46] Shekleton JA, Rogers NL, Rajaratnam SM. Searching for the daytime impairments of primary insomnia. Sleep Medicine Reviews. 2010;**14**(1):47-60. DOI: 10.1016/j.smrv.2009.06.001

[47] Edinger JD, Means MK, Carney CE, Krystal AD. Psychomotor performance deficits and their relation to prior nights' sleep among individuals with primary insomnia. Sleep. 2008;**31**(5):599-607. DOI: 10.1093/sleep/31.5.599

[48] Orff HJ, Drummond SP, Nowakowski S, Perils ML. Discrepancy between subjective symptomatology and objective neuropsychological performance in insomnia. Sleep. 2007;**30**(9):1205-1211. DOI: 10.1093/sleep/30.9.1205

[49] Boyle J, Trick L, Johnsen S, Roach J, Rubens R. Next-day cognition, psychomotor function, and driving-related skills following nighttime administration of eszopiclone. Human Psychopharmacology. 2008;**23**(5):385-397. DOI: 10.1002/hup.936

[50] Haimov I, Hanuka E, Horowitz Y. Chronic insomnia and cognitive functioning among older adults. Behavioral Sleep Medicine. 2008;**6**(1):32-54. DOI: 10.1080/15402000701796080

[51] Shekleton JA, Flynn-Evans EE, Miller B, Epstein LJ, Kirsch D, Brogna LA, et al. Neurobehavioral performance impairment in insomnia: Relationships with self-reported sleep and daytime functioning. Sleep. 2014;**37**(1):107-116. DOI: 10.5665/sleep.3318

[52] Fortier-BrochuE,Beaulieu-BonneauS, Ivers H, Morin CM. Insomnia and daytime cognitive performance: A meta-analysis. Sleep Medicine Reviews. 2012;**16**(1):83-94. DOI: 10.1016/j.smrv.2011.03.008

[53] Cellini N, de Zambotti M, Covassin N, Sarlo M, Stegagno L. Impaired off-line motor skills consolidation in young primary insomniacs. Neurobiology of Learning and Memory. 2014;**114**:141-147. DOI: 10.1016/j.nlm.2014.06.006

[54] Sandi C. Stress and cognition. Wiley Interdisciplinary Reviews: Cognitive Science. 2013;**4**(3):245-261. DOI: 10.1002/wcs.1222

[55] Calvo MG, Gutierrez-Garcia A. Cognition and stress. In: Fink G, editor. Stress: Concepts, Cognition, Emotion, and Behavior. San Diego, CA, USA: Academic Press; 2016. pp. 139-144. Available online: https://www.sciencedirect.com/science/article/pii/B9780128009512000169

[56] The American Physiological Association (APA). Stress in America™: Are Teens Adopting Adults' Stress Habits? was developed, reviewed and produced by the following team of experts. 2014 [Accessed: 13 January 2023]

[57] Tang YP, Shimizu E, Dube GR, Rampon C, Kerchner GA, Zhuo M, et al. Genetic enhancement of learning and memory in mice. Nature. 1999;**401**(6748):63-69. DOI: 10.1038/43432

[58] Riedel A, Stober F, Richter K, Fischer KD, Miettinen R, Budinger E. VGLUT3-immunoreactive afferents of the lateral septum: Ultrastructural evidence for a modulatory role of glutamate. Brain Structure & Function. 2013;**218**(1):295-301. DOI: 10.1007/s00429-012-0395-4

[59] Li XK, Tu B, Zhang XA, Xu W, Chen JH, Zhao GY, et al. Dysregulation of glutamine/glutamate metabolism in COVID-19 patients: A metabolism study in African population and mini meta-analysis. Journal of Medical Virology. 2023;**95**(1):e28150. DOI: 10.1002/jmv.28150

[60] Sonnewald U, Westergaard N, Schousboe A, Svendsen JS, Unsgard G, Petersen SB. Direct demonstration by [13C] NMR spectroscopy that glutamine from astrocytes is a precursor for GABA synthesis in neurons. Neurochemistry International. 1993;**22**(1):19-29. DOI: 10.1016/0197-0186(93)90064-c

[61] Petroff OA. GABA and glutamate in the human brain. The Neuroscientist. 2002;**8**(6):562-573. DOI: 10.1177/1073858402238515

[62] Schwartz RD, Mindlin MC. Inhibition of the GABA receptor-gated chloride ion channel in brain by noncompetitive inhibitors of the nicotinic receptor-gated cation channel. The Journal of Pharmacology and Experimental Therapeutics. 1988;**244**(3):963-970. ISSN (Linking): 0022-3565

[63] Roberts E, Frankel S. Gamma-aminobutyric acid in brain: Its formation from glutamic acid. The Journal of Biological Chemistry. 1950;**187**(1):55-63. ISSN (Linking): 0021-9258

[64] Roberts E, Eidelberg E. Metabolic and neurophysiological roles of gamma-aminobutyric acid. International Review of Neurobiology. 1960;**2**:279-332. DOI: 10.1016/s0074-7742(08)60125-7

[65] Bouche N, Lacombe B, Fromm H. GABA signaling: A conserved and ubiquitous mechanism. Trends in Cell Biology. 2003;**13**(12):607-610. DOI: 10.1016/j.tcb.2003.10.001

[66] Martin DL, Rimvall K. Regulation of gamma-aminobutyric acid synthesis in the brain. Journal of Neurochemistry. 1993;**60**(2):395-407. DOI: 10.1111/j.1471-4159.1993.tb03165.x

[67] Dionisio L, Jose De Rosa M, Bouzat C, Esandi MC. An intrinsic GABAergic system in human lymphocytes. Neuropharmacology. 2011;**60**(2-3):513-519. DOI: 10.1016/j.neuropharm.2010.11.007

[68] Foster JD, Kitchen I, Bettler B, Chen Y. GABAB receptor subtypesdifferentially modulate synaptic inhibition in the dentate gyrus to enhancegranule cell output. British Journal of Pharmacology. 2013;**168**:1808-1819. DOI: 10.1111/bph.12073

[69] Haeney CF, Kinney JW. Role of GABAB receptors in learning and memory and neurological disorders. Neurosci Behav Rev. 2016;**63**:1-28. DOI: 10.1016/j.neubiorev.2016.01.007

[70] Rashmi D, Zanan R, John S, Khandagale K, Nadaf A. Chapter 13 - g-aminobutyric acid (GABA): Biosynthesis, role, commercial production, and applications. Studies in Natural Products Chemistry. 2018;**57**:413-452. DOI: 10.1016/B978-0-444-64057-4.00013-2

[71] Gottesmann C. GABA mechanisms and sleep. Neuroscience. 2002;**111**:231-239. DOI: 10.1016/S0306-4522(02)00034-9

[72] Nemeroff CB. The Role of GABA in the Pathophysiology and Treatment of anxiety disorders. Psychopharmacology Bulletin. 2003;**37**:133-146

[73] Jie F, Yin G, Yang W, Yang M, Gao S, Lv J, et al. Stress in regulation of GABA amygdala system and relevance to neuropsychiatric diseases. Frontiers in Neuroscience. 2018;**12**:562. DOI: 10.3389/fnins.2018.00562

[74] Nuss P. Anxiety disorders and GABA neurotransmission: A disturbance of modulation. Neuropsychiatric Disease and Treatment. 2015;**11**:165-175. DOI: 10.2147/NDT.S58841

[75] Riemann D, Nissen C, Palagini L, Otte A, Perlis ML, Spiegelhalder K. The neurobiology, investigation, and treatment of chronic insomnia. Lancet Neurology. 2015;**14**:547-558. DOI: 10.1016/S1474-4422(15)00021-6

[76] Lichstein KL, Nau SD, Wilson NM, Aguillard RN, Lester KW, Bush AJ, et al. Psychological treatment of hypnotic-dependent insomnia in a primarily older adult sample. Behaviour Research and Therapy. 2013;**51**:787-796

[77] Lozano-Soldevilla D, ter Huurne N, Cools R, Jensen O. GABAergic modulation of visual gamma and alpha oscillations and its consequences for working memory performance. Current Biology. 2014;**24**(24):2878-2887. DOI: 10.1016/j.cub.2014.10.017

[78] Schmidt-Wilcke T, Fuchs E, Funke K, Vlachos A, Muller-Dahlhaus F, Puts NAJ. GABA-from inhibition to cognition: Emerging concepts. The Neuroscientist. 2018;**24**(5):501-515. DOI: 10.1177/1073858417734530

[79] Torta DM, Castelli L, Zibetti M, Lopiano L, Geminiani G. On the role of dopamine replacement therapy in decision-making, working memory, and reward in Parkinson's disease: Does the therapy-dose matter? Brain and Cognition. 2009;**71**(2):84-91. DOI: 10.1016/j.bandc.2009.04.003

[80] Jutras MJ, Buffalo EA. Synchronous neural activity and memory formation. Current Opinion in Neurobiology.

2010;**20**(2):150-155. DOI: 10.1016/j.conb.2010.02.006

[81] Hollnagel JO, Maslarova A, Haq RU, Heinemann U. GABAB receptor dependent modulation of sharp wave-ripple complexes in the rat hippocampus in vitro. Neuroscience Letters. 2014;**574**:15-20. DOI: 10.1016/j.neulet.2014.04.045

[82] Dubrovina NI, Zinov'ev DR. Contribution of GABA receptors to extinction of memory traces in normal conditions and in a depression-like state. Neuroscience and Behavioral Physiology. 2008;**38**(8):775-779. DOI: 10.1007/s11055-008-9045-y

[83] Nakagawa Y, Iwasaki T, Ishima T, Kimura K. Interaction between benzodiazepine and GABA-A receptors in state-dependent learning. Life Sciences. 1993;**52**(24):1935-1945. DOI: 10.1016/0024-3205(93)90634-f

[84] Pontes A, Zhang Y, Hu W. Novel functions of GABA signaling in adult neurogenesis. Frontiers in Biology (Beijing). 2013;**8**(5):496-507. DOI: 10.1007/s11515-013-1270-2

[85] Kreisel T, Frank MG, Licht T, et al. Dynamic microglial alterations underlie stress-induced depressive-like behavior and suppressed neurogenesis Molecular Psychiatry. 2014;19(6):699-709. Doi: 10.1038/mp.2013.155

[86] Nunan R, Sivasathiaseelan H, Khan D, Zaben M, Gray W. Microglial VPAC1R mediates a novel mechanism of neuroimmune-modulation of hippocampal precursor cells via IL-4 release. Glia. 2014;**62**(8):1313-1327. DOI: 10.1002/glia.22682

[87] Fatemi SH, Reutiman TJ, Folsom TD, Rooney RJ, Patel DH, Thuras PD. mRNA and protein levels for GABAAalpha4, alpha5, beta1 and GABABR1 receptors are altered in brains from subjects with autism. Journal of Autism and Developmental Disorders. 2010;**40**(6):743-750. DOI: 10.1007/s10803-009-0924-z

[88] Enticott PG, Kennedy HA, Rinehart NJ, Tonge BJ, Bradshaw JL, Fitzgerald PB. GABAergic activity in autism spectrum disorders: An investigation of cortical inhibition via transcranial magnetic stimulation. Neuropharmacology. 2013;**68**:202-209. DOI: 10.1016/j.neuropharm.2012.06.017

[89] DeLorey TM, Sahbaie P, Hashemi E, Homanics GE, Clark JD. Gabrb3 gene deficient mice exhibit impaired social and exploratory behaviors, deficits in non-selective attention and hypoplasia of cerebellar vermal lobules: A potential model of autism spectrum disorder. Behavioural Brain Research. 2008;**187**(2):207-220. DOI: 10.1016/j.bbr.2007.09.009

[90] Alroughani R, Akhtar S, Ahmed SF, Behbehani R, Al-Abkal J, Al-Hashel J. Incidence and prevalence of pediatric onset multiple sclerosis in Kuwait: 1994-2013. Journal of the Neurological Sciences. 2015;**353**(1-2):107-110. DOI: 10.1016/j.jns.2015.04.025

[91] Demakova EV, Korobov VP, Lemkina LM. Determination of gamma-aminobutyric acid concentration and activity of glutamate decarboxylase in blood serum of patients with multiple sclerosis. Klin Lab Diagnostic. 2003;**4**:15-17

[92] Garjani A, Middleton RM, Hunter R, Tuite-Dalton KA, Coles A, Dobson R, et al. COVID-19 is associated with new symptoms of multiple sclerosis that are prevented by disease modifying therapies. Multiple Sclerosis and Related Disorders. 2021;**52**:102939. DOI: 10.1016/j.msard.2021.102939

[93] Zhang B, Vogelzang A, Miyajima M, Sugiura Y, Wu Y, Chamoto K, et al. B cell-derived GABA elicits IL-10(+) macrophages to limit anti-tumor immunity. Nature. 2021;**599**(7885):471-476

[94] Tian J, Chau C, Hales TG, Kaufman DL. GABA(A) receptors mediate inhibition of T cell responses. Journal of Neuroimmunology. 1999;**96**(1):21-28. DOI: 10.1016/s0165-5728(98)00264-1

[95] Prud'Homme GJ, Glinka Y, Hasilo C, Paraskevas S, Li X, Wang Q. GABA protects human islet cells against the deleterious effects of immunosuppressive drugs and exerts immunoinhibitory effects alone. Transplantation. 2013;**96**(7):616-623. DOI: 10.1097/TP.0b013e31829c24be

[96] Tian J, Lu Y, Zhang H, Chau CH, Dang HN, Kaufman DL. Gamma-aminobutyric acid inhibits T cell autoimmunity and the development of inflammatory responses in a mouse type 1 diabetes model. Journal of Immunology. 2004;**173**(8):5298-5304. DOI: 10.4049/jimmunol.173.8.5298

[97] Wang Y, Feng D, Liu G, Luo Q, Xu Y, Lin S, et al. Gamma-aminobutyric acid transporter 1 negatively regulates T cell-mediated immune responses and ameliorates autoimmune inflammation in the CNS. Journal of Immunology. 2008;**181**(12):8226-8236. DOI: 10.4049/jimmunol.181.12.8226

[98] Beales PE, Hawa M, Williams AJ, Albertini MC, Giorgini A, Pozzilli P. Baclofen, a gamma-aminobutyric acid-b receptor agonist, delays diabetes onset in the non-obese diabetic mouse. Acta Diabetologica. 1995;**32**(1):53-56. DOI: 10.1007/BF00581047

[99] Tian J, Dang H, Wallner M, Olsen R, Kaufman DL. Homotaurine, a safe blood–brain barrier permeable GABAA-R-specific agonist, ameliorates disease in mouse models of multiple sclerosis. Scientific Reports. 2018;**8**(1):16555. DOI: 10.1038/s41598-018-32,733-3

[100] Tian J, Dang H, O'Laco KA, Song M, Tiu BC, Gilles S, et al. Homotaurine Treatment Enhances CD4(+) and CD8(+) Regulatory T Cell Responses and Synergizes with Low-Dose Anti-CD3 to Enhance Diabetes Remission in Type 1 Diabetic Mice. Immunohorizons. 2019;**3**(10):498-510. DOI: 10.4049/immunohorizons.1900019

[101] Bhandage AK, Jin Z, Korol SV, Shen Q, Pei Y, Deng Q, et al. GABA regulates release of inflammatory cytokines from peripheral blood mononuclear cells and CD4(+) T Cells and Is Immunosuppressive in Type 1 Diabetes. Ebio Medicine. 2018;**30**:283-294. DOI: 10.1016/j.ebiom.2018.03.019

[102] Vabret N, Britton GJ, Gruber C, Hegde S, Kim J, Kuksin M, et al. Immunology of COVID-19: Current State of the Science. Immunity. 2020;**52**(6):910-941. DOI: 10.1016/j.immuni.2020.05.002

[103] Januzi L, Poirier JW, Maksoud MJE, Xiang YY, Veldhuizen RAW, Gill SE, et al. Autocrine GABA signaling distinctively regulates phenotypic activation of mouse pulmonary macrophages. Cellular Immunology. 2018;**332**:7-23. DOI: 10.1016/j.cellimm.2018.07.001

[104] Forstera B, Castro PA, Moraga-Cid G, Aguayo LG. Potentiation of Gamma Aminobutyric Acid Receptors (GABAAR) by Ethanol: How are inhibitory receptors affected? Frontiers in Cellular Neuroscience. 2016;**10**:114. DOI: 10.3389/fncel.2016.00114

[105] Paul AM, Branton WG, Walsh JG, Polyak MJ, Lu JQ, et al. GABA transport

and neuroinflammation are coupled in multiple sclerosis: regulation of the GABA transporter-2 by Ganaxolone. Neuroscience. 2014;**273**:24-38. DOI: 10.1016/j.neuroscience.2014.04.037

[106] Fu CY, He XY, Li XF, Zhang X, Huang ZW, Li J, et al. Nefiracetam Attenuates Pro-Inflammatory Cytokines and GABA Transporter in Specific Brain Regions of Rats with Post-Ischemic Seizures. Cellular Physiology and Biochemistry. 2015;**37**(5):2023-2031. DOI: 10.1159/000438562

[107] Su J, Yin J, Qin W, Sha S, Xu J, Jiang C. Role for pro-inflammatory cytokines in regulating expression of GABA transporter type 1 and 3 in specific brain regions of kainic acid-induced status epilepticus. Neurochemical Research. 2015;**40**(3):621-627. DOI: 10.1007/s11064-014-1504-y

[108] Hernandez-Rabaza V, Cabrera-Pastor A, Taoro-Gonzalez L, Gonzalez-Usano A, Agusti A, Balzano T, et al. Neuroinflammation increases GABAergic tone and impairs cognitive and motor function in hyperammonemia by increasing GAT-3 membrane expression. Reversal by sulforaphane by promoting M2 polarization of microglia. Journal of Neuroinflammation. 2016;**13**(1):83. DOI: 10.1186/s12974-016-0549-z

[109] Huang T, Zhang Y, Wang C, Gao J. Propofol reduces acute lung injury by up-regulating gamma-aminobutyric acid type a receptors. Experimental and Molecular Pathology. 2019;**110**:104295. DOI: 10.1016/j.yexmp.2019.104295

[110] Mahmoud K, Ammar A. Immunomodulatory effects of anesthetics during thoracic surgery. Anesthesiology Research Practise. 2011;**2011**:317410. DOI: 10.1155/2011/317410

[111] Pan CF, Shen MY, Wu CJ, Hsiao G, Chou DS, Sheu JR. Inhibitory mechanisms of gabapentin, an antiseizure drug, on platelet aggregation. The Journal of Pharmacy and Pharmacology. 2007;**59**(9):1255-1261. DOI: 10.1211/jpp.59.9.0010

[112] Lin KH, Lu WJ, Wang SH, Fong TH, Chou DS, Chang CC, et al. Characteristics of endogenous gamma-aminobutyric acid (GABA) in human platelets: Functional studies of a novel collagen glycoprotein VI inhibitor. Journal of Molecular Medicine (Berlin, Germany). 2014;**92**(6):603-614. DOI: 10.1007/s00109-014-1140-7

[113] Hottz ED, Azevedo-Quintanilha IG, Palhinha L, Teixeira L, Barreto EA, Pao CRR, et al. Platelet activation and platelet-monocyte aggregate formation trigger tissue factor expression in patients with severe COVID-19. Blood. 2020;**136**(11):1330-1341. DOI: 10.1182/blood.2020007252

[114] Tian J, Middleton B, Kaufman DL. GABA(A)-Receptor Agonists Limit Pneumonitis and Death in Murine Coronavirus-Infected Mice. Viruses. 2021;**13**(6):966. DOI: 10.3390/v13060966

[115] Khanolkar A, Fulton RB, Epping LL, Pham NL, Tifrea D, Varga SM, et al. T cell epitope specificity and pathogenesis of mouse hepatitis virus-1-induced disease in susceptible and resistant hosts. Journal of Immunology. 2010;**185**(2):1132-1141. DOI: 10.4049/jimmunol.0902749

[116] Krystal JH, D'Souza DC, Sanacora G, Goddard AW, Charney DS. Current perspectives on the pathophysiology of schizophrenia, depression, and anxiety disorders. The Medical Clinics of North America. 2001;**85**(3):559-577. DOI: 10.1016/s0025-7125(05)70329-1

[117] Morinushi T, Masumoto Y, Kawasaki H, Takigawa M. Effect on electroencephalogram of chewing flavored gum. Psychiatry and Clinical Neurosciences. 2000;**54**(6):645-651. DOI: 10.1046/j.1440-1819.2000.00772.x

[118] Abdou AM, Higashiguchi S, Horie K, Kim M, Hatta H, Yokogoshi H. Relaxation and immunity enhancement effects of gamma-aminobutyric acid (GABA) administration in humans. BioFactors. 2006;**26**(3):201-208. DOI: 10.1002/biof.5520260305

[119] Tomasi TB, Gray HM. Structure and function of immunoglobulin A. Progress in Allergy. 1972;**16**:81-213

[120] Asim M, Jiang S, Yi L, Chen W, Sun L, Zhao L. Glutamine is required for red-spotted grouper nervous necrosis virus replication via replenishing the tricarboxylic acid cycle. Virus Research. 2017;**227**:245-248. DOI: 10.1016/j.virusres.2016.11.007

[121] Kalyanaraman B. Reactive oxygen species, proinflammatory and immunosuppressive mediators induced in COVID-19: Overlapping biology with cancer. RSC Chemical Biology. 2021;**2**(5):1402-1414. DOI: 10.1039/d1cb00042j

[122] Kumar P, Osahon O, Vides DB, Hanania N, Minard CG, Rajagopal V, et al. Severe glutathione deficiency, oxidative stress and oxidant, damage in adults hospitalized with COVID-19: Implication, for GlyNAC (Glycine and N-Acetylcysteine) supplementation. Antioxidants. 2022;**11**:50. DOI: 10.3390/antiox11010050

[123] Yowtak J, Wang J, Kim HY, Lu Y, Chung K, Chung JM. Effect of antioxidant treatment on spinal GABA neurons in a neuropathic pain model in the mouse. Pain. 2013;**154**(11):2469-2476. DOI: 10.1016/j.pain.2013.07.024

[124] Ludewig B, Jaggi M, Dumrese T, Brduscha-Riem K, Odermatt B, Hengartner H. Hypercholesterolemia exacerbates virus-induced immunopathologic liver disease via suppression of antiviral cytotoxic T cell responses. Journal of Immunology. 2001;**166**(5):3369-3376. DOI: 10.4049/jimmunol.166.5.3369

[125] Wu Q, Zhou L, Sun X, Yan Z, Hu C, Wu J, et al. Altered lipid metabolism in recovered SARS patients twelve years after infection. Scientific Reports. 2017;**7**:9110. DOI: 10.1038/s41598-017-09536-z

[126] Nguyen A, Guedan A, Mousnier A, Swieboda D, Zhang Q, Horkai D, et al. Host lipidome analysis during rhinovirus replication in HBECs identifies potential therapeutic targets. Journal of Lipid Research. 2018;**59**(9):1671-1684. DOI: 10.1194/jlr.M085910

[127] Xu K, Nagy PD. RNA virus replication depends on enrichment of phosphatidylethanolamine at replication sites in subcellular membranes. Proceedings of the National Academy Science USA. 2015;**112**:E1782-E1791

[128] Grieb P, Swiatkiewicz M, Prus K, Rejdak K. Hypoxia may be a determinative factor in COVID-19 progression. Current Research Pharmacological Drug Discovery. 2021;**2**:100030. DOI: 10.1016/j.crphar.2021.100030

[129] Hannun YA, Obeid LM. Sphingolipids and their metabolism in physiology and disease. Nature Reviews. Molecular Cell Biology. 2018;**19**(3):175-191. DOI: 10.1038/nrm.2017.107

[130] Chakinala RC, Khatri A, Gupta K, Koike K, Epelbaum O. Sphingolipids in COPD. European Respiratory Review. 2019;**28**(154). DOI: 10.1183/16000617.0047-2019

[131] Yin Y, Xu L, Porter NA. Free radical lipid peroxidation: Mechanisms and analysis. Chemical Reviews. 2011;**111**(10):5944-5972. DOI: 10.1021/cr200084z

[132] Fruhwirth GO, Loidl A, Hermetter A. Oxidized phospholipids: From molecular properties to disease. Biochimica et Biophysica Acta, Molecular Basis of Disease. 2007;**1772**(7):718-736. DOI: 10.1016/j.bbadis.2007.04.009

[133] Kinnunen PKJ, Kaarniranta K, Mahalka A. Protein oxidized phospholipid interactions in cellular signaling for cell death: From biophysics to clinical correlations. Biochimica et Biophysica Acta. 2012;**1818**(10):2446-2455. DOI: 10.1016/j.bbamem.2012.04.008

[134] Gracanin M, Hawkins CL, Pattison DI, Davies MJ. Singlet-oxygen-mediated amino acid and protein oxidation: Formation of tryptophan peroxides and decomposition products. Free Radical Biology & Medicine. 2009;**47**(1):92-102. DOI: 10.1016/j.freeradbiomed.2009.04.015

[135] Zarkovic N, Cipak A, Jaganjac M, Borovic S, Zarkovic K. Pathophysiological relevance of aldehydic protein modifications. Journal of Proteomics. 2013;**92**:239-247. DOI: 10.1016/j.jprot.2013.02.004

[136] Ayala A, Munoz MF, Arguelles S. Lipid peroxidation: Production, metabolism, and signaling mechanisms of malondialdehyde and 4-hydroxy-2-nonenal. Oxidative Medical Cell Longevity. 2014;**2014**:360438. DOI: 10.1155/2014/360438

[137] Orioli M, Aldini G, Beretta G, Facino RM, Carini M. LC-ESI-MS/MS determination of 4-hydroxy-trans-2-nonenal Michael adducts with cysteine and histidine-containing peptides as early markers of oxidative stress in excitable tissues. Journal of Chromatography. B, Analytical Technologies in the Biomedical and Life Sciences. 2005;**827**(1):109-118. DOI: 10.1016/j.jchromb.2005.04.025

[138] Dringen R. Metabolism and functions of glutathione in brain. Progress in Neurobiology. 2000;**62**(6):649-671. DOI: 10.1016/s0301-0082(99)00060-x

[139] Pastore A, Federici G, Bertini E, Piemonte F. Analysis of glutathione: Implication in redox and detoxification. Clinica Chimica Acta. 2003;**333**(1):19-39. DOI: 10.1016/s0009-8981(03)00200-6

[140] Pastore A, Tozzi G, Gaeta LM, Giannotti A, Bertini E, Federici G, et al. Glutathione metabolism and antioxidant enzymes in children with Down syndrome. Journal of Peadiatric. 2003;**142**(5):583-585. DOI: 10.1067/mpd.2003.203

[141] Espinosa JM. Down Syndrome and COVID-19: A Perfect Storm? Cell Reports in Medicine. 2020;**1**(2):100019. DOI: 10.1016/j.xcrm.2020.100019

[142] Zhu Y, Carvey PM, Ling Z. Age-related changes in glutathione and glutathione-related enzymes in rat brain. Brain Research. 2006;**1090**(1):35-44. DOI: 10.1016/j.brainres.2006.03.063

[143] Poli G, Schaur RJ, Siems WG, Leonarduzzi G. 4-hydroxynonenal: A membrane lipid oxidation product of medicinal interest. Medicinal Research Reviews. 2008;**28**(4):569-631. DOI: 10.1002/med.20117

[144] Alary J, Gueraud F, Cravedi JP. Fate of 4-hydroxynonenal in vivo: Disposition and metabolic pathways. Molecular Aspects of Medicine.

2003;**24**(4-5):177-187. DOI: 10.1016/s0098-2997(03)00012-8

[145] Castegna A, Lauderback CM, Mohmmad-Abdul H, Butterfield DA. Modulation of phospholipid asymmetry in synaptosomal membranes by the lipid peroxidation products, 4-hydroxynonenal and acrolein: Implications for Alzheimer's disease. Brain Research. 2004;**1004**(1-2):193-197. DOI: 10.1016/j.brainres.2004.01.036

[146] LoPachin RM, Gavin T, Geohagen BC, Das S. Neurotoxic mechanisms of electrophilic type-2 alkenes: Soft interactions described by quantum mechanical parameters. Toxicological Sciences. 2007;**98**(2):561-570. DOI: 10.1093/toxsci/kfm127

[147] Vander Jagt DL, Hunsaker LA, Vander Jagt TJ, Gomez MS, Gonzales DM, Deck LM, et al. Inactivation of glutathione reductase by 4-hydroxynonenal and other endogenous aldehydes. Biochemical Pharmacology. 1997;**53**(8):1133-1140

[148] Carbone DL, Doorn JA, Kiebler Z, Ickes BR, Petersen DR. Modification of heat shock protein 90 by 4-hydroxynonenal in a rat model of chronic alcoholic liver disease. The Journal of Pharmacology and Experimental Therapeutics. 2005;**315**(1):8-15. DOI: 10.1124/jpet.105.088088

[149] Roede JR, Jones DP. Reactive species and mitochondrial dysfunction: Mechanistic significance of 4-hydroxynonenal. Environmental and Molecular Mutagenesis. 2010;**51**(5):380-390. DOI: 10.1002/em.20553

[150] Honzatko A, Brichac J, Murphy TC, Reberg A, Kubatova A, Smoliakova IP. Enantioselective metabolism of trans-4-hydroxy-2-nonenalbybrainmitochondria. Free Radical Biology & Medicine. 2005;**39**(7):913-924. DOI: 10.1016/j.freeradbiomed.2005.05.010

[151] Crabb DW, Galli A, Fischer M, You M, et al. Molecular mechanisms of alcoholic fatty liver: Role of peroxisome proliferator-activated receptor alpha. Alcohol. 2004;**34**(1):35-38. DOI: 10.1016/j.alcohol.2004.07.005

[152] Zheng R, Dragomir AC, Mishin V, Richardson JR, Heck DE, Laskin DL, et al. Differential metabolism of 4-hydroxynonenal in liver, lung and brain of mice and rats. Toxicology and Applied Pharmacology. 2014;**279**(1):43-52. DOI: 10.1016/j.taap.2014.04.026

[153] Corradi M, Pignatti P, Manini P, Andreoli R, Goldoni M, Poppa M, et al. Comparison between exhaled and sputum oxidative stress biomarkers in chronic airway inflammation. The European Respiratory Journal. 2004;**24**(6):1011-1017. DOI: 10.1183/09031936.04.00002404

[154] Stopforth A, Burger BV, Crouch AM, Sandra P. Urinalysis of 4-hydroxynonenal, a marker of oxidative stress, using stir bar sorptive extraction-thermal desorption-gas chromatography/mass spectrometry. Journal of Chromatography. B, Analytical Technologies in the Biomedical and Life Sciences. 2006;**834**(1-2):134-140. DOI: 10.1016/j.jchromb.2006.02.038

[155] Esterbauer H, Zollner H, Lang J. Metabolism of the lipid peroxidation product 4-hydroxynonenal by isolated hepatocytes and by liver cytosolic fractions. The Biochemical Journal. 1985;**228**(2):363-373. DOI: 10.1042/bj2280363

[156] Dianzani MU. 4-hydroxynonenal from pathology to physiology. Molecular Aspects of Medicine. 2003;**24**(4-5):263-272. DOI: 10.1016/s0098-2997(03)00021-9

[157] Curzio M, Torrielli MV, Giroud JP, Esterbauer H, Dianzani MU. Neutrophil chemotactic responses to aldehydes. Research Communication in Chemical Pathology and Pharmacology. 1982;**36**(3):463-476

[158] Paradisi L, Panagini C, Parola M, Barrera G, Dianzani MU. Effects of 4-hydroxynonenal on adenylate cyclase and 5′-nucleotidase activities in rat liver plasma membranes. Chemico-Biological Interactions. 1985;**53**(1-2):209-217. DOI: 10.1016/s0009-2797(85)80097-1

[159] Rossi MA, Garramone A, Dianzani MU. Stimulation of phospholipase C activity by 4-hydroxynonenal; influence of GTP and calcium concentration. International Journal of Tissue Reactions. 1988;**10**(5):321-325

[160] Camandola S, Poli G, Mattson MP. The lipid peroxidation product 4-hydroxy-2,3-nonenal increases AP-1-binding activity through caspase activation in neurons. Journal of Neurochemistry. 2000;**74**(1):159-168. DOI: 10.1046/j.1471-4159.2000.0740159.x

[161] Cajone F, Bernelli-Zazzera A. The action of 4-hydroxynonenal on heat shock gene expression in cultured hepatoma cells. Free Radical Research Communications. 1989;**7**(3-6):189-194. DOI: 10.3109/10715768909087941

[162] Spycher S, Tabataba-Vakili S, O'Donnell VB, Palomba L, Azzi A. 4-hydroxy-2,3-trans-nonenal induces transcription and expression of aldose reductase. Biochemical and Biophysical Research Communications. 1996;**226**(2):512-516. DOI: 10.1006/bbrc.1996.1386

[163] Basu-Modak S, Luscher P, Tyrrell RM. Lipid metabolite involvement in the activation of the human heme oxygenase-1 gene. Free Radical Biology & Medicine. 1996;**20**(7):887-897. DOI: 10.1016/0891-5849(95)02182-5

[164] Liu RM, Shi MM, Giulivi C, Forman HJ. Quinones increase gamma-glutamyl transpeptidase expression by multiple mechanisms in rat lung epithelial cells. The American Journal of Physiology. 1998;**274**(3):L330-L336. DOI: 10.1152/ajplung.1998.274.3.L330

[165] Siems W, Grune T. Intracellular metabolism of 4-hydroxynonenal. Molecular Aspects of Medicine. 2003;**24**(4-5):167-175. DOI: 10.1016/s0098-2997(03)00011-6

[166] Subramaniam R, Roediger F, Jordan B, Mattson MP, Keller JN, Waeg G, et al. The lipid peroxidation product, 4-hydroxy-2-trans-nonenal, alters the conformation of cortical synaptosomal membrane proteins. Journal of Neurochemistry. 1997;**69**(3):1161-1169. DOI: 10.1046/j.1471-4159.1997.69031161.x

[167] Shi Q, Vaillancourt F, Cote V, Fahmi H, Lavigne P, Afif H, et al. Alterations of metabolic activity in human osteoarthritic osteoblasts by lipid peroxidation end product 4-hydroxynonenal. Arthritis Research & Therapy. 2006;**8**(6):R159. DOI: 10.1186/ar2066

[168] Arunachalam G, Sundar IK, Hwang JW, Yao H, Rahman I. Emphysema is associated with increased inflammation in lungs of atherosclerosis-prone mice by cigarette smoke: Implications in comorbidities of COPD. Journal of Inflammation. 2010;7:34. DOI: 10.1186/1476-9255-7-34

[169] Zarkovic K. 4-hydroxynonenal and neurodegenerative diseases. Molecular Aspects of Medicine. 2003;**24**(4-5):293-303. DOI: 10.1016/s0098-2997(03)00024-4

[170] Bennaars-Eiden A, Higgins L, Hertzel AV, Kapphahn RJ, Ferrington DA, Bernlohr DA. Covalent modification of epithelial fatty acid-binding protein by 4-hydroxynonenal in vitro and in vivo. Evidence for a role in antioxidant biology. The Journal of Biological Chemistry. 2002;**277**(52):50693-50,702. DOI: 10.1074/jbc.M209493200

[171] Rahman I, van Schadewijk AA, Crowther AJ, Hiemstra PS, Stolk J, MacNee W, et al. 4-Hydroxy-2-nonenal, a specific lipid peroxidation product, is elevated in lungs of patients with chronic obstructive pulmonary disease. American Journal of Respiratory and Critical Care Medicine. 2002;**166**(4):490-495. DOI: 10.1164/rccm.2110101

[172] Dickinson DA, Forman HJ. Glutathione in defense and signaling: Lessons from a small thiol. Annals of the New York Academy of Sciences. 2002;**973**:488-504. DOI: 10.1111/j.1749-6632.2002.tb04690.x

[173] Zhang H, Liu H, Dickinson DA, Liu RM, Postlethwait EM, Laperche Y, et al. gamma-Glutamyl transpeptidase is induced by 4-hydroxynonenal via EpRE/Nrf2 signaling in rat epithelial type II cells. Free Radical Biology & Medicine. 2006;**40**(8):1281-1292. DOI: 10.1016/j.freeradbiomed.2005.11.005

[174] Malone PE, Hernandez MR. 4-Hydroxynonenal, a product of oxidative stress, leads to an antioxidant response in optic nerve head astrocytes. Experimental Eye Research. 2007;**84**(3):444-454. DOI: 10.1016/j.exer.2006.10.020

[175] Yang Y, Sharma R, Sharma A, Awasthi S, Awasthi YC. Lipid peroxidation and cell cycle signaling: 4-hydroxynonenal, a key molecule in stress mediated signaling. Acta Biochemica Pol. 2003;**50**(2):319-336

[176] Schmidt H, Grune T, Muller R, Siems WG, Wauer RR. Increased levels of lipid peroxidation products malondialdehyde and 4-hydroxynonenal after perinatal hypoxia. Pediatric Research. 1996;**40**(1):15-20. DOI: 10.1203/00006450-199,607,000-00003

[177] Grune T et al. Increased levels of 4-hydroxynonenal modified proteins in plasma of children with autoimmune diseases. Free Radical Biology & Medicine. 1997;**23**(3):357-360. DOI: 10.1016/s0891-5849(96)00586-2

[178] Lovell MA, Markesbery WR. Oxidative damage in mild cognitive impairment and early Alzheimer's disease. Journal of Neuroscience Research. 2007;**85**(14):3036-3040. DOI: 10.1002/jnr.21346

[179] Zhong Z, Zeng T, Xie K, Zhang C, Chen J, Bi Y, et al. Elevation of 4-hydroxynonenal and malondialdehyde modified protein levels in cerebral cortex with cognitive dysfunction in rats exposed to 1-bromopropane. Toxicology. 2013;**306**:16-23. DOI: 10.1016/j.tox.2013.01.022

[180] Bradley MA, Markesbery WR, Lovell MA. Increased levels of 4-hydroxynonenal and acrolein in the brain in preclinical Alzheimer disease. Free Radical Biology & Medicine. 2010;**48**(12):1570-1576. DOI: 10.1016/j.freeradbiomed.2010.02.016

[181] Pedersen WA, Fu W, Keller JN, Markesbery WR, Appel S, Smith RG, et al. Protein modification by the lipid peroxidation product 4-hydroxynonenal in the spinal cords of amyotrophic lateral sclerosis patients. Annals of Neurology. 1998;**44**(5):819-824. DOI: 10.1002/ana.410440518

[182] Fleuranceau-Morel P, Barrier L, Fauconneau B, Piriou A, Huguet F. Origin

of 4-hydroxynonenal incubation-induced inhibition of dopamine transporter and Na+/K+ adenosine triphosphate in rat striatal synaptosomes. Neursoci Lett. 1999;**277**(2):91-94. DOI: 10.1016/s0304-3940(99)00652-7

[183] Shin Y, White BH, Uh M, Sidhu A. Modulation of D1-like dopamine receptor function by aldehydic products of lipid peroxidation. Brain Research. 2003;**968**(1):102-113. DOI: 10.1016/s0006-8993(02)04279-8

[184] Moreau C, Devos D, Brunaud-Danel V, Defebvre L, Perez T, Destee A, et al. Elevated IL-6 and TNF-alpha levels in patients with ALS: Inflammation or hypoxia? Neurology. 2005;**6**(12):1958-1960. DOI: 10.1212/01.wnl.0000188907.97339.76

[185] Blanc EM, Kelly JF, Mark RJ, Waeg G, Mattson MP. 4-Hydroxynonenal, an aldehydic product of lipid peroxidation, impairs signal transduction associated with muscarinic acetylcholine and metabotropic glutamate receptors: Possible action on G alpha(q/11). Journal of Neurochemistry. 1997;**69**(2):570-578. DOI: 10.1046/j.1471-4159.1997.69020570.x

[186] Re G, Azzimondi G, Lanzarini C, Bassein L, Vaona I, Guarnieri C. Plasma lipoperoxidative markers in ischaemic stroke suggest brain embolism. European Journal of Emergency Medicine. 1997;**4**(1):5-9

[187] Newcombe J, Li H, Cuzner ML. Low density lipoprotein uptake by macrophages in multiple sclerosis plaques: Implications for pathogenesis. Neuropathology and Applied Neurobiology. 1994;**20**(2):152-162. DOI: 10.1111/j.1365-2990.1994.tb01174.x

[188] Stoy N, Mackay GM, Forrest CM, Christofides J, Egerton M, Stone TW, et al. Tryptophan metabolism and oxidative stress in patients with Huntington's disease. Journal of Neurochemistry. 2005;**93**(3):611-623. DOI: 10.1111/j.1471-4159.2005.03070.x

[189] Mark RJ, Keller JN, Kruman I, Mattson MP. Basic FGF attenuates amyloid beta-peptide-induced oxidative stress, mitochondrial dysfunction, and impairment of Na+/K + -ATPase activity in hippocampal neurons. Brain Research. 1997;**756**(1-2):205-214. DOI: 10.1016/s0006-8993(97)00196-0

[190] Eichenbaum H. Hippocampus: Cognitive processes and neural representations that underlie declarative memory. Neuron. 2004;**44**(1):109-120. DOI: 10.1016/j.neuron.2004.08.028

[191] Lisman J, Buzsaki G, Eichenbaum H, Nadel L, Ranganath C, Redish AD. Viewpoints: How the hippocampus contributes to memory, navigation and cognition. Nature Neuroscience. 2017;**20**(11):1434-1447. DOI: 10.1038/nn.4661

[192] Taki Y, Hashizume H, Thyreau B, Sassa Y, Takeuchi H, Wu K, et al. Sleep duration during weekdays affects hippocampal gray matter volume in healthy children. NeuroImage. 2012;**60**(1):471-475. DOI: 10.1016/j.neuroimage.2011.11.072

[193] Kreutzmann JC, Havekes R, Abel T, Meerlo P. Sleep deprivation and hippocampal vulnerability: Changes in neuronal plasticity, neurogenesis and cognitive function. Neuroscience. 2015;**309**:173-190. DOI: 10.1016/j.neuroscience.2015.04.053

[194] Klein R, Soung A, Sissoko C, Nordvig A, Canoll P, Mariani M, et al. COVID-19 induces neuroinflammation and loss of hippocampal neurogenesis. Research Sequence. 2021;**2021**:1031

[195] Liu Y, Xu G, Sayre LM. Carnosine inhibits (E)-4-hydroxy-2-nonenal-induced protein cross-linking: Structural characterization of carnosine-HNE adducts. Chemical Research in Toxicology. 2003;**16**(12):1589-1597. DOI: 10.1021/tx034160a

[196] Guiotto A, Calderan A, Ruzza P, Borin G. Carnosine and carnosine-related antioxidants: A review. Current Medicinal Chemistry. 2005;**12**(20):2293-2315. DOI: 10.2174/0929867054864796

[197] The National Institutes of Health (NIH). Vitamin C. Fact Sheet for Health Porfessionals. Office of Dietary Supplements (ODS). Vitamin C - Health Professional Fact Sheet (nih.gov). 2021 [Accessed: 17 January 2023]

[198] National Institutes of Health (NIH). Vitamin E. Fact Sheet for Health Porfessionals. Office of Dietary Supplements (ODS). Vitamin E - Health Professional Fact Sheet (nih.gov). 2021 [Accessed: 17 January 2023]

[199] Bassett IB, Pannowitz DL. Barnetson RSA comparative study of tea-tree oil versus benzoylperoxide in the treatment of acne. The Medical Journal of Australia. 1990;**153**(8):455-458. DOI: 10.5694/j.1326-5377.1990.tb126150.x

[200] Al-Sarraf H. Transport of 14C-gamma-aminobutyric acid into brain, cerebrospinal fluid and choroid plexus in neonatal and adult rats. Brain Research Development. 2002;**139**(2):121-129

[201] Yoto A, Murao S, Motoki M, Yokoyama Y, Horie N, Takeshima K, et al. Oral intake of gamma-aminobutyric acid affects mood and activities of central nervous system during stressed condition induced by mental tasks. Amino Acids. 2012;**43**(3):1331-1337. DOI: 10.1007/s00726-011-1206-6

[202] Tu J, Jin Y, Zhuo J, Cao X, Liu G, Du H, et al. Exogenous GABA improves the antioxidant and anti-aging ability of silkworm (Bombyx mori). Food Chemistry. 2022;**383**:132400. DOI: 10.1016/j.foodchem.2022.132400